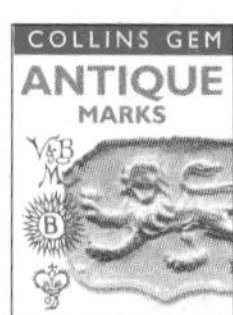
COLLINS GEM
ANTIQUE
MARKS

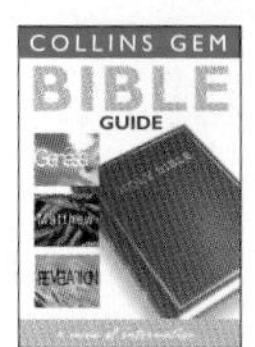
COLLINS GEM
BIBLE
GUIDE

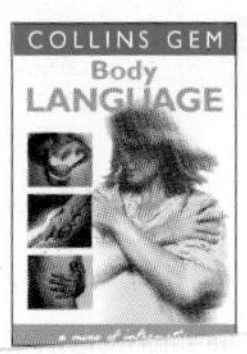
COLLINS GEM
Body
LANGUAGE

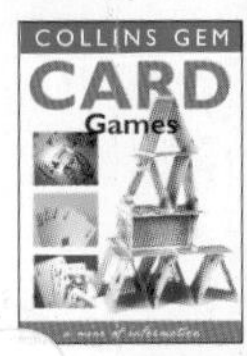
COLLINS GEM
CARD
Games

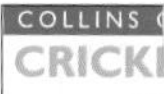
COLLINS G
CRICK

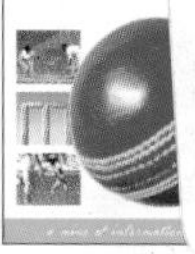

D1150058

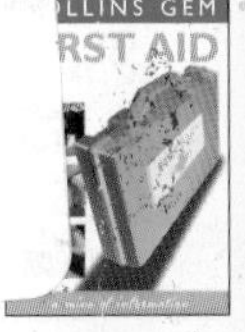
LLINS GEM
RST AID

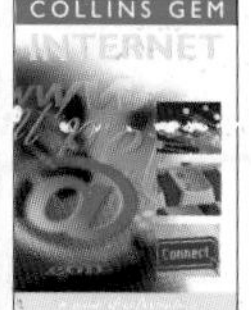
COLLINS GEM
INTERNET
Connect

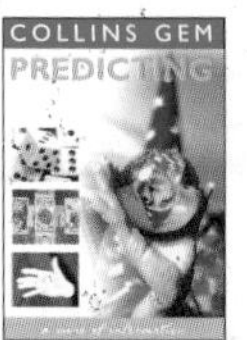
COLLINS GEM
PREDICTING

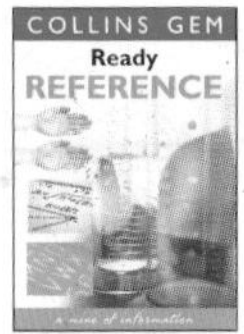
COLLINS GEM
Ready
REFERENCE

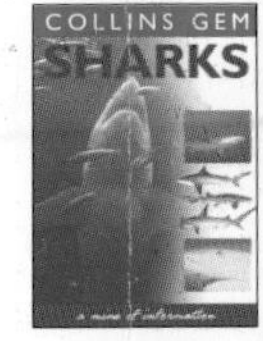
COLLINS GEM
SHARKS

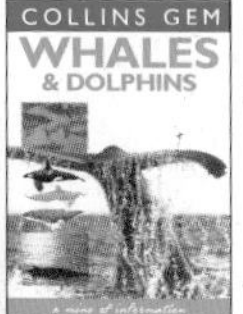
COLLINS GEM
WHALES
& DOLPHINS

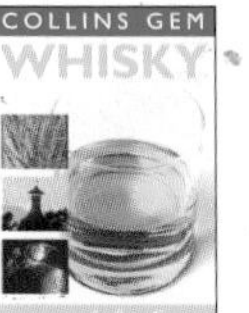
COLLINS GEM
WHISKY

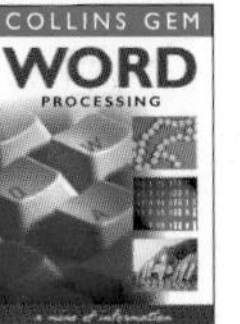
COLLINS GEM
WORD
PROCESSING

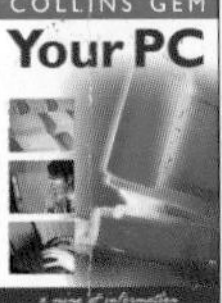
COLLINS GEM
Your PC

COLLINS GEM

CALORIE
Counter

HarperCollinsPublishers

This book has been compiled with the assistance of hundreds of brand-name manufacturers

HarperCollins Publishers
Westerhill Road, Bishopbriggs, Glasgow G64 2QT

First published 1984
Sixth edition published 1999
This edition published 2000

Reprint 10 9 8 7 6 5 4 3 2 1

ISBN 0 00 472470–4

Printed in Italy by Amadeus S.p.A.

PREFACE TO THE SEVENTH EDITION

Since its first publication in 1984, the *Collins Gem Calorie Counter* has firmly established itself as one of the most successful and popular reference guides available for weight watchers.

The text for this edition has been completely revised and updated. Included is data on the amount of Calories contained in a wide range of branded foods, as well as figures for the amount of protein, carbohydrate, fat and dietary fibre in the products covered. Doctors and nutritionists agree that combining these ingredients in the correct proportions is essential to ensure a healthy diet.

The inclusion of this information makes the *Collins Gem Calorie Counter* more than ever the ideal companion for the health-conscious shopper.

CONTENTS

Introduction 7

Useful Tables 15

- Weights and measures 16
- Average hourly Calorie requirement by activity 17
- Desirable weight of adults: small frame 18
- Desirable weight of adults: medium frame 19
- Desirable weight of adults: large frame 20
- Daily Calories for maintenance of desirable weight 21

Alphabetical listing of foods and their nutrients 23

INTRODUCTION

For many years, doctors and successful dieters alike have acknowledged that the healthiest and most effective form of weight loss is to combine a Calorie-controlled diet with regular exercise. Now that the body's metabolism is understood more fully, the informed dieter and health-conscious eater wants to know not only the Calorie content of food but also its composition.

The body can be compared to an engine, and the 'fuel' it uses is food. About half the energy provided by food is used to keep the body functioning normally; the other half is taken up by activity such as work and recreation. Generally speaking, active people use more energy and, therefore, need to eat more to meet their energy requirements. If a person consumes more energy than he or she expends, the excess will be stored by the body as fat, and the person will put on weight. Conversely, if a person consumes less energy than he or she expends the extra energy will be taken from the body's fat stores, and the person will lose weight.

The energy provided by food and burnt up by the body is generally measured in Calories, also called kilocalories (kcal). It has been calculated that one pound of body fat is equal to 3500 Calories, so for every pound required to be lost, 3500 Calories must be burnt up or cut out of the diet over several days. On page 13 there is a table which gives the average number of Calories used in an hour taking part in certain activities. However, the rate at which the body uses up Calories varies from person to person, and depends on many factors such as a person's age, sex and general state of fitness, as well as the composition of their diet.

The food that we eat is made up of three major kinds of nutrients: *proteins*, *carbohydrates* and *fats*. It also provides the body with vitamins and minerals; these are called micronutrients because they are required in much smaller quantities. Nutrients all have important functions within the body.

Proteins are the building bricks of the human body. The cells of our bones, muscles, skin, nails, hair and every other tissue are made up of proteins. Many vital fluids, such as blood, enzymes and hormones, also contain proteins. There is an enormous variety of different kinds of protein, each made up of a special combination of components called amino acids.

The protein in our food is broken down into its component amino acids by the digestive system, and new proteins are synthesized by the body. The best sources of protein in the diet are meat, fish, eggs, milk and other dairy products, corn, lentils and other pulses. The protein obtained from animal sources contains more amino acids than protein from plants. Vegans, therefore, have to eat a wide variety of foods in order to ensure that their diet includes the full complement of amino acids.

Nutritionists recommend that protein represents 10% of the body's daily energy intake. This means that if a person consumes about 2400 Calories a day, 240 of those Calories should be provided by the protein in their food. One gram of protein provides about 4 Calories, so that person needs to consume about 60 grams of protein a day. Many people eat more protein than this, and there is little evidence to suggest that eating too much protein is a health risk. However, a diet low in protein is harmful, particularly to the young who are still growing.

Carbohydrates are made up of different kinds of simple sugars, such as glucose. The scientific name for the sugar that we add to our food is sucrose; one molecule or unit of sucrose is made up of two units of glucose. Carbohydrates can be divided into two different categories. The first category, which we will simply call *carbohydrates*, are known as *available carbohydrates* because the body can obtain energy from them. The second category, usually called *dietary fibres*, are known as *unavailable carbohydrates* because they are indigestible.

Available carbohydrates are important sources of energy for the body. They are broken down by the digestive system into the individual simple sugars; then they can be metabolized immediately to release energy, or they can be converted into fat and put into the body's energy stores. Starch is a form of carbohydrate, and starchy foods – such as wheat, rice, pulses and potatoes – are a good source of carbohydrates. Carbohydrates are also found in fruit and vegetables. Honey, sugar, sweets and sweetened soft drinks contain very high levels of carbohydrates, but they provide the body with virtually no other nutrients. For this reason, energy from these sources is sometimes referred to as 'empty calories'.

Although the body can obtain energy from a diet that contains no carbohydrates, they are still an important part of the diet, not least because foods rich in carbohydrates are usually good sources of micronutrients. For example, grains provide B vitamins, and fruit is an important source of vitamin C. Nutritionists recommend that 50% of the body's energy requirements are derived from carbohydrates. If a person consumes 2400 Calories a day, 1200 of those Calories should be provided by carbohydrates in their food. One gram of carbohydrate provides about 4 Calories, so that person should eat about 300 grams of carbohydrates a day.

Unavailable carbohydrates, or **dietary fibre**, cannot be broken down by the digestive system. Dietary fibre adds bulk to food and contributes to the 'full' feeling after a meal. Although it does not contain any nutrients it is an essential part of the diet and it has a number of beneficial effects, especially assisting the regular and comfortable evacuation of the bowels. Certain kinds of dietary fibre, such as oat bran, are believed to lower levels of cholesterol in the blood. Foods that contain high levels of dietary fibre are, anyway, usually good sources of other nutrients and micronutrients. They include wheat bran and bran cereals, dried fruits, nuts, pulses, and leafy green vegetables.

The average UK diet provides only about 12 grams of

dietary fibre a day. Nutritionists recommend that this figure should be nearer 30 grams. If the intake of dietary fibre is increased too rapidly it may cause flatulence and diarrhoea. A very high consumption of fibre may impede the absorption of certain vital minerals.

Fats in food are the perennial enemy of the dieter. Fat has a very high energy value: 1 gram of fat provides 9 Calories; this is more than twice the calorific value of 1 gram of protein or of carbohydrate. The fat obtained from food is only broken down and used as energy when other sources of energy – carbohydrate and protein – have been exhausted. If all the fat in the diet is not converted into energy, it is simply laid down in the body's fat stores. A high intake of fats will, therefore, cause weight gain.

Vegetable oils, dripping, lard, butter, margarine, cream and nuts are all high in fat. Some meats also have a high fat content, but this can usually be reduced by trimming away the visible areas of fat before or after cooking. Fats obtained from animal sources, such as butter and cream, have been associated with an increased risk of coronary heart disease and of cancer if they are consumed in large quantities. Oils obtained from plants do not have this property, and certain vegetable and fish oils are thought to actively reduce the risk of heart disease.

Fat represents about 40% of the total energy intake of the average UK diet. This figure is much higher than it needs to be for the body's requirements. The body needs fat as an energy store and for the formation of cell membranes and the protective sheath that surrounds nerves, as well as the synthesis of certain hormones and enzymes. Most fats can be synthesized from excess carbohydrate and protein, but there are special fats called essential fatty acids which must be obtained from the diet. In order to ensure that these substances are included in the diet, fat should represent at least 2% of the body's energy intake.

However, a diet this low in fat would be unpalatable and difficult to prepare; nutritionists recommend that fat provides about 20% of the daily intake. This means that if a person consumes 2400 Calories a day, 480 of those Calories should be provided by fat in their food. Since 1 gram of fat provides 9 Calories, that person should eat about 53 grams of fat a day.

Among the tables on the following pages are those for desirable weights according to sex, height and frame. These will help to give the dieter a realistic target. Anyone considering trying to lose a lot of weight should consult their doctor, and those just keen not to overdo it should remember that the best way to lose weight – or to maintain a healthy weight – is to eat a balanced diet, to eat in moderation and to take regular exercise.

The foods in this book are listed in **bold type** in strict alphabetical order in the left-hand column of each page. Therefore **Crunchy Nut Cornflakes** will come after **Crunchie** which itself follows **Crunch Cakes**. The name of the manufacturer (of branded foods) is given in the second column. The energy value in Calories, the protein, carbohydrate, fat and dietary fibre contents per 100 gram or 100 millilitre are given in the third, fourth, fifth, sixth and seventh columns, respectively. The cross reference ***see individual brands/flavours/types***, e.g. under **Buns**, indicates that data for a particular foodstuff will be listed elsewhere, in this example under **Chelsea Buns, Currant Buns, Hot Cross Buns**, etc. Values for unbranded foods (listed in ***bold italic type***) have been obtained from *The Composition of Foods* (5th edition, 1991) and *Vegetables, Herbs and Spices* (supplement, 1991), and have been reproduced by permission of Controller of Her Majesty's Stationery Office.

The publishers are grateful to all the manufacturers who gave information on their products. The list of foods included is as up to date as it was possible to make it, but it should be remembered that new food products are frequently put on the market and existing ones withdrawn, so it has not been possible to include everything. If you cannot find a particular food here, you can still, however, obtain guideline figures by finding an equivalent product from one of the other manufacturers listed in the book.

USEFUL TABLES

Weights and measures

Imperial to Metric

1 ounce (oz) = 28.35 grams (g)
1 pound (lb) = 453.60 grams (g)
1 fluid ounce (fl oz) = 29.57 millilitres (ml)
1 pint = 0.568 litre

Metric to Imperial

100 grams (g) = 3.53 ounces (oz)
1 kilogram (kg) = 2.2 pounds (lb)
100 millilitres (ml) = 3.38 fluid ounces (fl oz)
1 litre = 1.76 pints

Average hourly Calorie requirement by activity

	Women	Men
Bowling	207	270
Cycling: moderate	192	256
hard	507	660
Dancing: ballroom	264	352
Domestic work	153	200
Driving	108	144
Eating	84	112
Gardening: active	276	368
Golf	144	192
Ironing	120	160
Office work: active	120	160
Rowing	600	800
Running: moderate	444	592
hard	692	900
Sewing and knitting	84	112
Sitting at rest	84	112
Skiing	461	600
Squash	461	600
Swimming: moderate	230	300
hard	480	640
Table tennis	300	400
Tennis	336	448
Typing	108	144
Walking: moderate	168	224

Desirable weight of adults: small frame

Height (without shoes)			Weight range						Height (without shoes)			Weight range					
ft	in	m	st	lb	st	lb	kg	kg	ft	in	m	st	lb	st	lb	kg	kg
5	1	1.55	8	0	8	8	50.8	54.4	4	8	1.42	6	8	7	10	41.7	44.5
5	2	1.58	8	3	8	12	52.2	56.3	4	9	1.45	6	10	7	3	42.6	45.8
5	3	1.60	8	6	9	0	53.5	57.2	4	10	1.47	6	12	7	6	43.6	47.2
5	4	1.63	8	9	9	3	54.9	58.5	4	11	1.50	7	1	7	9	44.9	48.5
5	5	1.65	8	12	9	7	56.3	60.3	5	0	1.52	7	4	7	12	46.3	49.9
5	6	1.68	9	2	9	11	58.1	62.1	5	1	1.55	7	7	8	1	47.6	51.3
5	7	1.70	9	6	10	1	59.9	64.0	5	2	1.58	7	10	8	4	49.0	52.6
5	8	1.73	9	10	10	5	61.7	65.8	5	3	1.60	7	13	8	7	50.4	54.0
5	9	1.75	10	0	10	10	63.5	68.0	5	4	1.63	8	2	8	11	51.7	55.8
5	10	1.78	10	4	11	0	65.3	69.9	5	5	1.65	8	6	9	1	53.5	57.6
5	11	1.80	10	8	11	4	67.1	71.7	5	6	1.68	8	10	9	5	55.3	59.4
6	0	1.83	10	12	11	8	69.0	73.5	5	7	1.70	9	0	9	9	57.2	61.2
6	1	1.85	11	2	11	13	70.8	75.8	5	8	1.73	9	4	10	0	59.0	63.5
6	2	1.88	11	6	12	3	72.6	77.6	5	9	1.75	9	8	10	4	60.8	65.3
6	3	1.91	11	10	12	7	74.4	79.4	5	10	1.78	9	12	10	8	62.6	67.1

Desirable weight of adults: medium frame

Height (without shoes)			Weight range					
ft	in	m	st	lb	st	lb	kg	kg
5	1	1.55	8	6	9	3	53.5	58.5
5	2	1.58	8	9	9	7	54.9	60.3
5	3	1.60	8	12	9	10	56.3	61.7
5	4	1.63	9	1	9	13	57.6	63.1
5	5	1.65	9	4	10	3	59.0	64.9
5	6	1.68	9	8	10	7	60.8	66.8
5	7	1.70	9	12	10	12	62.6	69.0
5	8	1.73	10	2	11	2	64.4	70.8
5	9	1.75	10	6	11	6	66.2	72.6
5	10	1.78	10	10	11	11	68.0	74.8
5	11	1.80	11	0	12	2	69.9	77.1
6	0	1.83	11	4	12	7	71.7	79.4
6	1	1.85	11	8	12	12	73.5	81.7
6	2	1.88	11	13	13	3	75.8	83.9
6	3	1.91	12	4	13	8	78.0	86.2

Height (without shoes)			Weight range					
ft	in	m	st	lb	st	lb	kg	kg
4	8	1.42	6	12	7	9	43.6	48.5
4	9	1.45	7	0	7	12	44.5	49.9
4	10	1.47	7	3	8	1	45.8	51.3
4	11	1.50	7	6	8	4	47.2	52.6
5	0	1.52	7	9	8	7	48.5	54.0
5	1	1.55	7	12	8	10	49.9	55.3
5	2	1.58	8	1	9	0	51.3	57.2
5	3	1.60	8	4	9	4	52.6	59.0
5	4	1.63	8	8	9	9	54.4	61.2
5	5	1.65	8	12	9	13	56.3	63.1
5	6	1.68	9	2	10	3	58.1	64.9
5	7	1.70	9	6	10	7	59.9	66.7
5	8	1.73	9	10	10	11	61.7	68.5
5	9	1.75	10	0	11	1	63.5	70.3
5	10	1.78	10	4	11	5	65.3	72.1

Desirable weight of adults: large frame

Height (without shoes)			Weight range						Height (without shoes)			Weight range					
ft	in	m	st	lb	st	lb	kg	kg	ft	in	m	st	lb	st	lb	kg	kg
5	1	1.55	9	0	10	1	57.2	64.0	4	8	1.42	7	6	8	7	47.2	54.0
5	2	1.58	9	3	10	4	58.5	65.3	4	9	1.45	7	8	8	10	48.1	55.3
5	3	1.60	9	6	10	8	59.9	67.1	4	10	1.47	7	11	8	13	49.4	56.7
5	4	1.63	9	9	10	12	61.2	69.0	4	11	1.50	8	0	9	2	50.8	58.1
5	5	1.65	9	12	11	2	62.6	70.8	5	0	1.52	8	3	9	5	52.2	59.4
5	6	1.68	10	2	11	7	64.4	73.0	5	1	1.55	8	6	9	8	53.5	60.8
5	7	1.70	10	7	11	12	66.7	75.3	5	2	1.58	8	9	9	12	54.9	62.6
5	8	1.73	10	11	12	2	68.5	77.1	5	3	1.60	8	13	10	2	56.7	64.4
5	9	1.75	11	1	12	6	70.3	78.9	5	4	1.63	9	3	10	6	58.5	66.2
5	10	1.78	11	5	12	11	72.1	81.2	5	5	1.65	9	7	10	10	60.3	68.0
5	11	1.80	11	10	13	2	74.4	83.5	5	6	1.68	9	11	11	0	62.1	69.9
6	0	1.83	12	0	13	7	76.2	85.7	5	7	1.70	10	1	11	4	64.0	71.7
6	1	1.85	12	5	13	12	78.5	88.0	5	8	1.73	10	5	11	9	65.8	73.9
6	2	1.88	12	10	14	3	80.7	90.3	5	9	1.75	10	9	12	0	67.6	76.2
6	3	1.91	13	0	14	8	82.6	92.5	5	10	1.78	10	13	12	5	69.4	78.5

Daily Calories for maintenance of desirable weight

Calculated for a moderately active life. If you are very active add 50 Calories; if your life is sedentary subtract 75 Calories.

Weight			Age 18–35		Age 35–55		Age 55–75	
st	lb	kg	Men	Women	Men	Women	Men	Women
7	1	44.9		1700		1500		1300
7	12	49.9	2200	1850	1950	1650	1650	1400
8	9	54.9	2400	2000	2150	1750	1850	1550
9	2	58.1		2100		1900		1600
9	6	59.9	2550	2150	2300	1950	1950	1650
10	3	64.9	2700	2300	2400	2050	2050	1800
11	0	69.9	2900	2400	2600	2150	2200	1850
11	11	74.8	3100	2550	2800	2300	2400	1950
12	8	79.8	3250		2950		2500	
13	5	84.8	3300		3100		2600	

ALPHABETICAL LISTING OF FOODS AND THEIR NUTRIENTS

Abbreviations used in the Tables

g	gram
kcal	kilocalorie
ml	millilitre
N	the nutrient is present in significant quantities but there is no accurate information on the amount
n/a	not available
Tr	trace (less than 0.1g present)

A

Product	*Brand*	*Calories kcal*	*Protein (g)*	*Carbo-hydrate (g)*	*Fat (g)*	*Dietary Fibre (g)*
Abbey Crunch Biscuits	McVitie's	479	6.1	73.1	18.0	2.6
Action Man Pasta Shapes in Tomato Sauce	Heinz	59.0	1.9	12.0	0.4	0.6
Advocaat		272	4.7	28.4	6.3	nil
Aero Chocolate Drinks, all flavours	Nestlé	97.0	4.6	12.4	3.2	0.2
Aero Chocolate Orange	Chambourcy	211	6.1	27.4	8.6	0.1
Aero Milk Chocolate Mousse, per serving	Chambourcy	155	2.9	16.8	7.9	0.6

All amounts given per 100g/100ml unless otherwise stated

Product	*Brand*	*Calories kcal*	*Protein (g)*	*Carbo-hydrate (g)*	*Fat (g)*	*Dietary Fibre (g)*
Aero Peppermint Chocolate Mousse, per serving	Chambourcy	155	2.9	16.8	7.9	0.6
After Eight Mints	Nestlé Rowntree	419	2.5	72.4	13.3	1.0
After Eight White Chocolate Mints	Nestlé Rowntree	422	2.6	76.9	11.6	n/a
Alabama Chocolate Fudge Cake	McVitie's	373	4.4	61.5	12.5	0.8
Albert's Victorian Chutney	Baxters	151	0.9	36.2	0.3	1.0
Alfredo Pasta Choice as sold	Crosse & Blackwell	480	14.3	55.7	11.3	2.5
All-Bran Buds	Kellogg's	270	13.0	47.0	3.5	29.0
All-Bran Bite Size	Kellogg's	290	15.0	48.0	4.0	22.0
All-Bran Plus	Kellogg's	270	13.0	45.0	4.0	29.0
All Day Breakfast Platter, each	Birds Eye	710	25.0	42.0	49.0	5.8

All Juice Lemonade	Cawston Vale	44.0	Tr	11.7	Tr	n/a
Allora	Cadbury	540	8.0	51.2	33.9	n/a
Almonds, flaked/ground		612	21.1	6.9	55.8	12.9
Almond Slice	Mr Kipling	375	6.8	57.7	13.0	n/a
Alpen	Weetabix	364	10.2	65.5	6.8	7.6
no added sugar	Weetabix	363	12.6	62.1	7.2	7.8
Alphabites	Birds Eye	156	2.5	21.4	6.7	1.8
Amber Sugar Crystals	Tate & Lyle	398	Tr	99.9	nil	nil
Ambrosia Products: *see Rice, Sago, etc.*						
American Ginger Ale	Schweppes	22.0	nil	5.3	nil	n/a
American Hard Gums	Trebor Bassett	345	Tr	85.6	nil	nil
American Potato & Leek Chowder Soup of the World	Knorr	354	8.0	57.8	10.1	4.8
American Style BBQ Waffles	Boots Shapers	338	n/a	n/a	1.5	n/a
Anchovies canned in oil, drained		280	25.2	nil	19.9	nil
Anchovy Essence	Burgess	150	13.3	nil	10.4	nil

All amounts given per 100g/100ml unless otherwise stated

Product	*Brand*	*Calories kcal*	*Protein (g)*	*Carbo-hydrate (g)*	*Fat (g)*	*Dietary Fibre (g)*
Anchovy Paste	Shippams	164	19.5	3.1	8.2	n/a
Angel Delight, as sold	Bird's					
Banana		490	2.5	72.0	21.0	nil
Butterscotch		475	2.4	73.5	19.0	nil
Chocolate		455	3.7	69.5	18.0	0.4
Forest Fruit		490	2.5	71.5	21.5	nil
Raspberry		490	2.5	72.0	21.0	nil
Strawberry		485	2.5	71.0	21.0	nil
Toffee		480	2.6	70.0	21.0	nil
Vanilla Ice Cream		490	2.5	71.5	21.5	nil
Angel Delight, sugar free, as sold	Bird's					
Banana Toffee		495	4.8	58.5	26.5	nil
Butterscotch		480	4.5	61.0	24.0	nil
Chocolate		450	6.3	56.5	22.0	0.6
Raspberry		465	4.8	59.5	26.5	nil
Strawberry		495	4.8	58.0	27.0	nil
Tangerine		495	4.8	58.0	27.0	0.9
Vanilla Ice Cream		500	4.8	59.5	27.0	nil

Angel Delight Chocolate Topples	Bird's	465	5.0	67.0	20.0	0.5
Angel Delight Strawberry Topples	Bird's	450	2.8	74.5	14.0	0.7
Angel Slice	Mr Kipling	404	3.1	53.5	17.5	n/a
Animal Bar	Nestlé Rowntree	513	5.8	63.6	26.1	n/a
Apple & Banana Bio Yogurt	Holland & Barrett	54.0	4.4	5.6	1.5	nil
Apple & Blackcurrant Fruit Burst	Del Monte	45.0	0.1	11.0	Tr	n/a
Apple & Blackberry Hot Cake	McVitie's	306	3.8	41.8	14.3	1.3
Apple & Blackberry with Custard Twinpot Yogurt	St Ivel Shape	50.0	4.7	6.8	0.1	0.2
Apple & Blackcurrant Drink	Quosh	72.0	Tr	16.6	Tr	n/a
	Robinsons	37.0	Tr	8.1	Tr	n/a
	Boots Shapers	2.0	n/a	n/a	Tr	n/a
Apple & Blackcurrant Fruit Pie Bars	Mr Kipling	373	3.5	57.1	14.2	n/a

All amounts given per 100g/100ml unless otherwise stated

Product	*Brand*	*Calories kcal*	*Protein (g)*	*Carbo-hydrate (g)*	*Fat (g)*	*Dietary Fibre (g)*
Apple & Blackcurrant Individual Pies	Mr Kipling	343	3.1	53.4	12.7	n/a
Apple & Blackcurrant Pies	Mr Kipling	346	3.5	54.4	12.6	n/a
Apple & Blackcurrant Special R ready to drink carton	Robinsons	4.2	Tr	0.7	Tr	n/a
Apple & Blackberry Yogurt	Boots Shapers	87.0	n/a	n/a	0.1	n/a
Apple & Cinnamon Oatso Simple	Quaker	358	8.0	68.0	5.5	2.5
Apple & Raisin Harvest Chewy Bar, each	Quaker	89.0	1.2	15.0	2.6	0.7
Apple & Sour Cherry Juice	Cawston Vale	44.0	0.1	10.8	Tr	n/a
Apple & Spice Yogurt	St Ivel Shape	57.0	5.3	7.7	0.2	0.2
Apple & Strawberry Juice	Copella	39.0	n/a	10.1	nil	Tr
Apple & Strawberry Juice Drink	Robinsons	88.0	Tr	21.0	Tr	Tr

Apple & Sultana Cereal Bar	Boots Shapers	317	n/a	n/a	11.0	n/a
Apple 'C'	Libby	47.0	Tr	11.7	Tr	nil
Apple Chutney		201	0.9	52.2	0.2	1.2
Apple Crumble	McVitie's	252	3.3	41.8	8.4	0.9
Apple Crush	Boots Shapers	8.0	n/a	n/a	Tr	n/a
	Jusoda	31.0	n/a	9.5	Tr	Tr
Apple Drink, Sparkling	St Clements	47.0	n/a	11.6	Tr	Tr
Apple Fruit Juice	Del Monte	47.0	0.3	10.8	Tr	n/a
Apple Hot 'n' Fruity Custard Pot, each	Bird's	174	1.6	32.5	4.1	0.2
Apple Jack Chews	Trebor Bassett	398	0.7	84.0	6.1	nil
Apple Juice	Britvic 55	46.0	Tr	11.0	Tr	n/a
	Copella	39.0	n/a	10.1	nil	Tr
unsweetened		38.0	0.1	9.9	0.1	Tr
Apple Juice Drink, as sold	Robinsons	87.0	Tr	20.0	Tr	n/a
ready to drink	Robinsons	46.0	Tr	11.0	Tr	n/a

All amounts given per 100g/100ml unless otherwise stated

Product	*Brand*	*Calories kcal*	*Protein (g)*	*Carbo-hydrate (g)*	*Fat (g)*	*Dietary Fibre (g)*
Apple Pashka	McVitie's	244	4.4	26.8	13.5	0.6
Apple Pies	McVitie's	235	2.8	35.3	9.6	0.9
Apple Rice Dessert	St Ivel	122	2.8	21.6	2.7	0.1
Apple Rings	Holland & Barrett	238	2.0	60.1	0.5	9.7
Apples, cooking						
raw, peeled		35.0	0.3	8.9	0.1	2.2
stewed with sugar		74.0	0.3	19.1	0.1	1.8
stewed without sugar		33.0	0.3	8.1	0.1	1.8
Apples, eating, average, raw		47.0	0.4	11.8	0.1	2.0
Apple Sauce	Heinz	61.0	0.3	14.5	0.2	1.4
Apple Strudel & Custard Twinpot Yogurt	St Ivel Shape	56.0	4.6	8.4	0.1	0.1
Apple Tango	Britvic	39.0	Tr	9.3	Tr	n/a
Low Calorie	Britvic	4.5	Tr	0.8	Tr	n/a

Apricot & Almond Frusli Bar, each	Jordans	556	2.0	21.3	4.3	1.6
Apricot & Chocolate Chip Cereal Bar	Boots Shapers	317	n/a	n/a	8.2	n/a
Apricot & Mango Extrafruit Yogurt	Ski	94.0	4.9	17.5	0.7	1.0
Apricot & Passionfruit Still Water	Boots Shapers	1.0	n/a	n/a	Tr	n/a
Apricot & Raisin Flapjacks	Mr Kipling	426	4.5	51.4	22.5	n/a
Apricot Cake Bar	Jacob's Vitalinea	377	4.1	66.5	10.5	0.9
Apricot Chutney	Sharwood	141	1.0	33.9	0.1	4.3
Apricot Fromage Frais	St Ivel Shape	69.0	6.9	7.0	1.2	Tr
Apricot Fruit Spread	Heinz Weight Watchers	110	0.3	27.2	nil	0.5
Apricot Halves in Syrup	Del Monte	78.0	0.4	18.5	0.2	n/a
	Libby	74.0	0.4	18.0	Tr	0.4

All amounts given per 100g/100ml unless otherwise stated

Product	Brand	Calories kcal	Protein (g)	Carbo-hydrate (g)	Fat (g)	Dietary Fibre (g)
Apricot Jam	Baxters	210	Tr	53.0	Tr	0.81
Apricot Muesli	Holland & Barrett	285	7.7	59.2	3.5	5.6
Apricots, raw		31.0	0.9	7.2	0.1	1.4
canned in syrup		63.0	0.4	16.1	0.1	1.2
canned in juice		34.0	0.5	8.4	0.1	1.2
Apricot Sucrose Free Jam	Dietade	260	0.3	64.4	Tr	nil
Apricot Yogurt Mousse	Boots Shapers	80.0	n/a	n/a	3.9	n/a
Aromat	Knorr	267	13.4	3.7	22.1	n/a
Artichoke, globe, raw		18.0	2.8	2.7	0.2	N
boiled		8.0	1.2	1.2	0.1	N
Artichoke, Jerusalem, boiled		41.0	1.6	10.6	0.1	N
Asparagus, raw		25.0	2.9	2.0	0.6	1.7
boiled		13.0	1.6	0.7	0.4	0.7
canned, drained		24.0	3.4	1.5	0.5	2.9

Asparagus Cup-A-Soup, per sachet	Batchelors	143	1.1	20.4	6.3	0.8
Assorted Jellies	Trebor Bassett	306	nil	81.6	nil	nil
Astros	Cadbury	470	4.8	73.1	17.3	nil
Aubergine, sliced, fried		302	1.2	2.8	31.9	2.9
Austrian Cream of Herb Soup of the World	Knorr	482	8.8	47.0	28.8	2.2
Autumn Vegetable Soup	Baxters	40.0	1.8	8.0	0.2	1.5
Avocado Pear, average		190	1.9	1.9	19.5	3.4

All amounts given per 100g/100ml unless otherwise stated

B

Product	*Brand*	*Calories kcal*	*Protein (g)*	*Carbo-hydrate (g)*	*Fat (g)*	*Dietary Fibre (g)*
Baby Button Sprouts	Ross	35.0	4.1	6.6	0.5	3.2
Baby Carrots	Birds Eye	22.0	0.8	4.6	Tr	2.0
Baby Sweetcorn: ***see Sweetcorn***						
Bacon & Mushroom filled pasta	Findus	90	3.0	12.5	2.5	1.1
Bacon & Tomato Filler	Primula	220	7.7	2.3	20.0	1.3
Bacon, collar joint						
lean & fat, boiled		325	20.4	nil	27.0	nil
lean only, boiled		191	26.0	nil	9.7	nil

All amounts given per 100g/100ml unless otherwise stated

Product	Brand	Calories kcal	Protein (g)	Carbo-hydrate (g)	Fat (g)	Dietary Fibre (g)
Bacon, gammon						
joint, lean & fat, boiled		269	24.7	nil	18.9	nil
joint, lean only, boiled		167	29.4	nil	5.5	nil
Bacon, rashers						
lean only, fried (average)		332	32.8	nil	22.3	nil
lean only, grilled (average)		292	30.5	nil	18.9	nil
back , lean & fat, fried		465	24.9	nil	40.6	nil
middle, lean & fat, fried		477	24.1	nil	42.3	nil
middle, lean & fat, grilled		416	24.9	nil	35.1	nil
streaky, lean & fat, fried		496	23.1	nil	44.8	nil
streaky, lean & fat, grilled		422	24.5	nil	36.0	nil
Bacon, Lettuce & Tomato Sandwiches, per pack	Boots Shapers	332	16.0	31.0	16.0	3.8
Bacon Supernoodles	Batchelors	480	10.3	63.9	20.7	3.4
Bacon Wheat Crunchies, Crispy	Golden Wonder	172	3.9	19.6	8.7	1.0

Food	Brand					
Baked Beans in tomato sauce		84.0	5.2	15.3	0.6	6.9
	Heinz	75.0	4.7	13.6	0.2	3.7
	HP	85.0	4.7	15.0	0.7	3.7
no added sugar	Heinz Weight Watchers	56.0	4.7	8.6	0.2	3.7
with reduced sugar		73.0	5.4	12.5	0.6	7.1
Baked Beans with Bacon	Heinz	91.0	6.0	12.9	1.7	3.0
Baked Beans with Chicken Nuggets	Heinz	104	6.6	12.4	3.1	3.2
Baked Beans with Pork Sausages	Heinz	89.0	5.5	11.2	2.5	2.6
Baked Beans with Vegetable Sausages	Heinz	102	5.6	12.1	3.5	2.9
Baked Potatoes, old, with flesh & skin		136	3.9	31.7	0.2	2.7
Bakers Yeast: ***see Yeast***						
Bakewell Slice	Mr Kipling	415	3.8	57.0	19.1	n/a
Bakewell Tart	McVitie's	396	5.0	48.9	20.4	0.7
	Mr Kipling	418	3.8	59.2	18.5	n/a

All amounts given per 100g/100ml unless otherwise stated

Product	Brand	Calories kcal	Protein (g)	Carbo-hydrate (g)	Fat (g)	Dietary Fibre (g)
Baking Powder		163	5.2	37.8	Tr	nil
Balti Cook-In-Sauce	Homepride	58.0	1.1	8.1	2.4	n/a
Balti Sizzle & Stir Sauce	Batchelors	116	1.3	6.3	9.5	2.9
Bamboo Shoots, canned		11.0	1.5	0.7	0.2	1.7
	Amoy	39.0	0.7	9.7	n/a	n/a
	Sharwood	6.0	0.8	0.3	0.2	1.6
Banana and Toffee Crisp	Mornflake	445	6.3	69.8	15.6	3.9
Banana Cake	California Cake & Cookie Ltd	409	3.2	63.0	16.0	0.7
Banana Chips	Holland & Barrett	511	1.0	59.9	31.4	1.1
	Whitworths	526	1.0	59.9	31.4	1.7
Banana Country Crisp	Jordans	439	7.6	66.2	16.0	6.1
Banana Crusha	Burgess	104	0.2	25.3	Tr	Tr
Banana Flavour Custard Dessert	Ambrosia	99.0	2.7	16.3	2.6	0.1

Banana Fromage Frais	St Ivel Shape	73.0	7.0	7.8	1.2	0.1
Banana Fudge Hot Crunch Pudding Mix	Bird's	445	5.4	75.0	14.0	0.8
Banana Napoli	Lyons Maid	95.0	1.7	10.5	5.1	n/a
Banana Nesquik	Nestlé	395	nil	97.3	0.5	nil
made up with whole milk	Nestlé	168	6.8	18.9	7.8	n/a
with semi-skimmed	Nestlé	155	6.8	24.9	3.4	nil
ready to drink	Nestlé	68.0	3.2	10.2	1.6	nil
Banana Nesquik Dessert	Nestlé	450	3.7	74.6	15.1	0.3
Bananas		95.0	1.2	23.2	0.3	3.1
Banana with Toffee Sauce Sponge Pudding	Heinz	291	2.7	48.8	9.4	0.7
Banoffee Corner House Cake	Lyons Cakes	399	3.2	50.6	19.2	n/a
Barbecue Beans	Heinz	82.0	4.9	14.9	0.3	4.0
Barbecue Beef & Tomato Cup-A-Soup , per sachet	Batchelors	116	1.6	20.1	3.2	0.7

All amounts given per 100g/100ml unless otherwise stated

Product	*Brand*	*Calories kcal*	*Protein (g)*	*Carbo-hydrate (g)*	*Fat (g)*	*Dietary Fibre (g)*
Barbecue Beef Supernoodles	Batchelors	478	9.9	63.6	20.7	3.4
Barbecue Beef Wotsits, per pack	Golden Wonder	110	1.5	11.7	6.3	0.3
Barbecue Coat and Cook, as sold	Homepride	407	10.4	51.5	17.0	n/a
Barbecue Cook-In-Sauce	Homepride	74.0	0.8	14.0	N	n/a
Barbecue 'Marinade in Minutes'	Knorr	302	4.5	67.1	1.7	n/a
Barbecue Pot Noodle	Golden Wonder	439	10.9	60.9	15.4	3.8
Barbecue Relish	Burgess	136	1.8	29.3	0.7	1.0
Barbecue Sauce		75.0	1.8	12.2	1.8	N
	Burgess	118	1.7	25.8	0.3	0.9
Barley Sugar	Cravens	385	Tr	96.3	nil	nil
	Trebor Bassett	389	nil	97.2	nil	nil
Basil & Oregano Sauce	Ragu	38.0	2.0	7.6	Tr	0.8

Basil Herb Cubes	Knorr	457	6.1	32.2	33.8	0.6
Basmati Rice	Uncle Ben's	343	9.0	75.5	0.6	n/a
	Whitworths	339	7.4	79.8	0.5	0.5
Bath Oliver	Jacob's	436	9.5	67.0	14.4	2.6
Bath Oliver Biscuits	Fortts	412	8.4	65.5	2.7	n/a
Battenburg Cake	Lyons Cakes	414	4.7	67.7	12.8	n/a
	Mr Kipling	398	6.2	67.4	11.5	n/a
Batter Mix, Quick	Whitworths	338	9.3	77.2	1.2	3.7
Bavarois Lemon Dessert	Chambourcy	160	2.4	22.7	6.6	Tr
Beanfeast (Batchelors): ***see individual flavours***						
Beans: ***see types***						
Beansprouts, mung, raw		31.0	2.9	4.0	0.5	5.6
boiled		25.0	2.5	2.8	0.5	1.3
canned		10.0	1.6	0.8	0.1	0.7
stir fried in oil		25.0	1.9	2.5	6.1	0.9
Beany Cheez Xtreme Dipz	Primula	282	12.6	22.6	15.6	N

All amounts given per 100g/100ml unless otherwise stated

Product	Brand	Calories kcal	Protein (g)	Carbo-hydrate (g)	Fat (g)	Dietary Fibre (g)
Beany Cheez Xtreme Sqeez	Primula	291	14.0	8.7	22.2	N
Beef						
brisket lean & fat, boiled		326	27.6	nil	23.9	nil
forerib, roast		349	22.4	nil	28.8	nil
mince, stewed		229	23.1	nil	15.2	nil
rump steak, lean & fat, fried		246	28.6	nil	14.6	nil
rump steak, lean & fat, grilled		218	27.3	nil	12.1	nil
rump steak, lean only, fried		190	30.8	nil	7.4	nil
rump steak, lean only, grilled		168	28.6	nil	6.0	nil
silverside, lean & fat, boiled		242	28.6	nil	14.2	nil
silverside, lean only, boiled		173	32.3	nil	4.9	nil
sirloin, lean & fat, roast		284	23.6	nil	21.1	nil
sirloin, lean only, roast		192	27.6	nil	9.1	nil
stewing steak, lean & fat, stewed		223	30.9	nil	11.0	nil
topside, lean & fat, roast		214	26.6	nil	12.0	nil
topside, lean only, roast		156	29.2	nil	4.4	nil
Beef & Kidney	Tyne Brand	97.0	10.5	2.0	5.2	n/a
Beef & Kidney Pie	Tyne Brand	154	8.7	13.3	8.1	n/a

Beef & Mushroom Pie	Tyne Brand	162	10.1	11.8	8.3	n/a
Beef & Potato Pie	Tyne Brand	191	7.1	22.2	8.2	n/a
Beef & Tomato Pot Noodle	Golden Wonder	408	11.8	56.7	14.8	3.6
Beef & Vegetable Pie	Tyne Brand	185	6.5	22.5	7.7	n/a
Beef & Vegetable Soup	Heinz Big Soups	45.0	2.4	7.3	0.7	0.9
Beef Bourguignon Casserole Mix, per pack	Colman's	119	1.9	25.6	0.7	n/a
Beef Broth	Heinz Big Soups	41.0	2.0	6.8	0.6	0.7
Beefburgers, fried		264	20.4	7.0	17.3	1.4
100%	Ross	293	17.0	nil	25.0	nil
100%, each	Birds Eye	125	6.5	0.3	11.0	nill
economy	Ross	255	13.6	9.9	18.1	0.4
original, each	Birds Eye	115	8.7	2.0	8.0	0.1
quarter-pounders, each	Birds Eye	200	17.5	4.0	12.7	0.2
Beef Casserole	Tyne Brand	93.0	6.2	6.5	4.7	n/a
Beef Chilli	Heinz Baked Bean Cuisine	85.0	4.6	10.8	2.6	1.7

All amounts given per 100g/100ml unless otherwise stated

Product	Brand	Calories kcal	Protein (g)	Carbo-hydrate (g)	Fat (g)	Dietary Fibre (g)
Beef Consomme	Baxters	16.0	2.4	1.1	0.1	nil
Beef Curry	Tyne Brand	98.0	5.5	9.2	4.3	n/a
as sold	Vesta	359	13.4	60.7	7.0	5.6
with rice, per pack	Birds Eye	525	26.0	80.0	11.0	3.1
Beef Dripping		891	Tr	Tr	99.0	nil
Beefeater Fast Fry Chips	McCain	132	2.2	23.0	3.5	n/a
Beefeater Oven Ready	McCain	115	2.0	27.5	4.1	n/a
Beef Goulash Casserole Mix, per pack	Colman's	119	2.0	27.0	0.2	n/a
Beef Grillsteaks, grilled, each	Birds Eye	205	14.0	3.0	15.0	0.1
Beef in Black Bean Sauce Readymeal	Uncle Ben's	85.0	6.3	8.1	3.0	n/a
Beef in Stout & Mash, per pack	Birds Eye	355	20.0	42.0	11.0	2.5

Beef Lasagne	Heinz Baked Bean Cuisine	90.0	5.1	11.5	2.6	1.2
Beef Lasagne	Heinz Weight Watchers	98.0	5.9	13.5	2.3	0.7
Beef Curry	Findus Red Box	140	5.4	18.3	4.9	1.0
Beef Risotto, as sold	Vesta	346	15.3	57.8	5.9	5.6
Beef Sausages: ***see Sausages, beef***						
Beef Savoury Rice	Batchelors	358	9.4	74.9	2.3	3.2
Beef Seasoning Dry Sauce Mix, per pack	Colman's	110	2.8	23.8	0.3	n/a
Beef Spread	Shippams	164	15.7	4.0	9.5	n/a
Beef Stew		120	9.7	4.6	7.2	0.7
	Tyne Brand	83.0	4.8	7.2	3.8	n/a
Beef Stew & Dumpling, per pack	Birds Eye	355	23.0	39.0	12.0	3.7
Beef Stock Cubes	Knorr	326	11.1	21.0	22.0	0.2

All amounts given per 100g/100ml unless otherwise stated

Product	*Brand*	*Calories kcal*	*Protein (g)*	*Carbo-hydrate (g)*	*Fat (g)*	*Dietary Fibre (g)*
Beef Stock Powder	Knorr	149	11.0	18.3	3.5	0.4
Beef Stroganoff Casserole Mix, per pack	Colman's	156	6.4	18.8	6.0	n/a
Beer						
bitter, canned		32.0	0.3	2.3	Tr	nil
bitter, draught		32.0	0.3	2.3	Tr	nil
bitter, keg		31.0	0.3	2.3	Tr	nil
mild, draught		25.0	0.2	1.6	Tr	nil
Beetroot, raw		36.0	1.7	7.6	0.1	2.8
boiled		46.0	2.3	9.5	0.1	2.3
pickled		28.0	1.2	5.6	0.2	2.5
pickled, all varieties	Baxters	30.0	1.5	6.0	Tr	1.2
Beetroot in Redcurrant Jelly	Baxters	167	0.7	43.9	Tr	0.9
Bengal Hot Chutney	Sharwood	200	0.5	48.7	0.3	1.1
Berry Fruits Crush	Boots Shapes	8.0	n/a	n/a	Tr	n/a
Berry Passion Bio Yogurt	St Ivel Shape	73.0	5.2	9.6	1.1	0.2

Best Burgers	Ross	298	12.7	4.2	25.6	0.2
Best English Mints	Cravens	387	Tr	96.1	0.2	nil
Big Breakfast, each	McDonald's	591	26.2	39.8	36.3	4.0
Bigga Processed Peas	Batchelors	66.0	5.6	10.1	0.3	4.0
Big Mac, each	McDonald's	493	26.7	44.0	22.9	5.5
Big Soups (Heinz): ***see individual flavours***						
Biscuits						
chocolate, full coated		524	5.7	67.4	27.6	2.9
digestive, chocolate		493	6.8	66.5	24.1	3.1
digestive, plain		471	6.3	68.6	20.9	4.6
sandwich		513	5.0	69.2	25.9	1.1
semi-sweet		457	6.7	74.8	16.6	2.1
short-sweet		469	6.2	62.2	23.4	1.5
Bisto It's So Easy Sauce, as sold	Centura					
Cracked Black Peppercorn		452	4.4	60.3	21.5	1.0
Garlic & Herb		413	3.7	65.0	15.4	1.1
Mild Mustard		420	6.5	57.6	18.1	1.2

Product	*Brand*	*Calories kcal*	*Protein (g)*	*Carbo-hydrate (g)*	*Fat (g)*	*Dietary Fibre (g)*
Bisto Cheese Sauce Granules, as sold	Centura	592	6.4	28.6	45.8	0.6
Bisto Chicken Gravy Granules, as sold	Centura	389	3.2	56.2	16.8	1.4
Bisto Curry Sauce Granules	Centura	164	1.4	13.4	11.6	n/a
Bisto Fuller Flavour Gravy Granules, as sold	Centura	317	3.8	66.7	4.2	0.8
Bisto Onion Gravy Granules, as sold	Centura	399	2.9	55.2	18.5	1.8
Bisto Original, made up	Centura	391	3.1	55.2	17.6	1.5
Bisto Parsley Sauce Granules, as sold	Centura	584	3.6	43.4	44.0	0.8
Bisto Vegetarian Granules, as sold	Centura	394	2.6	54.9	18.2	1.3
Bitter: ***see Beer***						

Bitter Lemon	Schweppes	33.9	Tr	8.2	nil	n/a
Black Bean & Vegetable Stir Fry Sauce	Uncle Ben's	50.0	1.8	9.0	0.7	n/a
Black Bean Sauce	Amoy	150	10.3	22.7	2.0	n/a
Straight to Wok	Amoy	139	2.0	32.0	0.3	n/a
Black Bean Stir Fry Mix, as sold	Crosse & Blackwell	375	10.8	65.3	7.6	2.8
Black Bean Stir Fry Sauce	Sharwood	90.0	0.3	19.9	1.3	1.2
Blackberries, raw		25.0	0.9	5.1	0.2	6.6
stewed with sugar		56.0	0.7	13.8	0.2	5.2
stewed without sugar		21.0	0.8	4.4	0.2	5.6
Black Cherries in Syrup	Libby	73.0	n/a	n/a	Tr	n/a
Black Cherry Crusha	Burgess	153	nil	37.1	nil	nil
Blackcherry Ripple Mousse, each	Fiesta	87.0	2.0	11.6	4.0	n/a
Black Cherry Yogurt	Boots Shapers	91.0	n/a	n/a	0.1	n/a
	Ski	95.0	5.1	17.3	1.1	nil

All amounts given per 100g/100ml unless otherwise stated

Product	*Brand*	*Calories kcal*	*Protein (g)*	*Carbo-hydrate (g)*	*Fat (g)*	*Dietary Fibre (g)*
Blackcurrant & Apple Drink	Boots Shapers	2.0	n/a	n/a	Tr	n/a
Blackcurrant & Apple Juice	Copella	50.0	n/a	12.5	nil	Tr
Blackcurrant & Liquorice	Cravens	404	0.6	91.4	4.1	nil
Blackcurrant Bio Stirred Yogurt	Ski	109	5.8	16.0	2.9	nil
Blackcurrant 'C'	Libby	54.0	Tr	13.5	Tr	nil
Blackcurrant Cheesecake	Eden Vale	261	2.8	38.8	11.6	n/a
	Heinz Weight Watchers	159	6.0	24.0	4.1	0.7
	McVitie's	296	4.5	31.9	17.1	0.7
Blackcurrant Cordial, as sold	Britvic	56.5	Tr	13.0	nil	n/a
BlackcurrantDessert Mousse	St Ivel Shape	55.0	3.8	3.7	2.3	0.2
Blackcurrant C-Vit	SmithKline Beecham	19.0	Tr	4.5	nil	n/a

Blackcurrant Fruit Spread	Heinz Weight Watchers	106	0.2	26.3	nil	0.9
Blackcurrant Jam	Baxters	210	Tr	53.0	Tr	1.3
Blackcurrant Juice Drink	Ribena	59.0	Tr	15.6	n/a	n/a
undiluted	Ribena	285	Tr	76.0	n/a	n/a
Blackcurrant Juice Ready to Drink Carton	Robinsons	59.0	Tr	14.4	Tr	n/a
Blackcurrant Party Cheesecake	McVitie's	295	4.4	33.8	16.1	0.8
Blackcurrant Sorbet	Del Monte	106	0.4	27.1	Tr	n/a
Blackcurrant Sparkling Water	Boots Shapers	1.0	n/a	n/a	Tr	n/a
Blackcurrants, raw		28.0	0.9	6.6	Tr	7.8
stewed with sugar		58.0	0.7	15.0	Tr	6.1
canned in juice		31.0	0.8	7.6	Tr	4.2
canned in syrup		72.0	0.7	18.4	Tr	3.6
Blackcurrant Sucrose Free Jam	Dietade	269	0.3	67.0	Tr	n/a

All amounts given per 100g/100ml unless otherwise stated

Product	*Brand*	*Calories kcal*	*Protein (g)*	*Carbo-hydrate (g)*	*Fat (g)*	*Dietary Fibre (g)*
Blackened Tandoori Chicken/ Roast Chicken Salad/ Barbecue Chicken 3-pack Sandwiches, per pack	Boots Shapers	432	26.0	46.0	16.0	5.4
Blackeye Beans, boiled		116	8.8	19.9	0.7	3.5
Black Forest Gateau	McVitie's	291	2.6	36.1	15.3	0.4
Black Forest Party Gateau	McVitie's	302	2.7	33.8	17.5	0.5
Black Jack Chews	Trebor Bassett	399	0.7	85.0	6.0	nil
Black Magic Assortment	Nestlé Rowntree	453	4.4	62.5	20.6	1.6
Black Pudding, fried		305	12.9	15.0	21.9	0.5
Black Treacle	Lyle's	290	1.7	64.0	nil	nil
Blended Autumn Vegetable Soup	Heinz	57.0	1.2	6.4	3.0	0.7
Blended Carrot & Coriander Soup	Heinz	52.0	0.7	6.2	2.7	0.6

Blended Leek & Bacon Soup	Heinz	54.0	1.9	5.0	2.9	0.5
Blended Mediterranean Tomato & Courgette Soup	Heinz	40.0	1.0	5.1	1.8	0.6
Blended Parsnip & Potato Soup	Heinz	57.0	1.1	6.4	3.0	0.9
Blended Red Pepper with Tomato Soup	Heinz	51.0	0.8	5.2	2.9	0.7
Bloater Paste	Shippams	171	17.2	2.5	10.4	n/a
Blue Band Margarine	Van den Bergh	658	0.1	0.1	73.0	nil
Blueberry & Blackberry Organic Jam	Baxters	252	Tr	63.0	Tr	1.4
Blueberry Napoli	Lyons Maid	104	1.8	12.7	5.2	n/a
Blue Cheese Dip, per pack	Boots Shapers	145	n/a	n/a	12.0	n/a
Blue Cheese Flavoured Low Fat Dressing	Heinz Weight Watchers	59.0	1.5	5.8	3.4	nil

All amounts given per 100g/100ml unless otherwise stated

Product	Brand	Calories kcal	Protein (g)	Carbo-hydrate (g)	Fat (g)	Dietary Fibre (g)
Blue Cheese Soured Cream Dip	St Ivel Shape	416	3.7	2.8	43.3	0.1
Blue Riband	Nestlé Rowntree	516	5.2	64.0	26.6	1.0
Blue Stilton Cheese: ***see Stilton***						
Boasters	McVitie's	547	6.3	54.8	33.1	1.8
Bodyline Natural Cottage Cheese	Eden Vale	85.0	14.0	4.4	1.5	nil
Bodyline Onion & Chive Cottage Cheese	Eden Vale	105	12.7	4.3	4.0	nil
Bodyline Pineapple Cottage Cheese	Eden Vale	97.0	11.6	5.3	3.5	0.2
Boiled Sweets		327	Tr	87.3	Tr	nil
Bolognese Beanfeast, per packet, as served	Batchelors	302	23.9	39.0	5.6	13.5
Bolognese Pasta Choice	Crosse & Blackwell	355	12.6	63.7	5.2	3.0

Bolognese Pot Pasta	Golden Wonder	349	17.7	59.8	4.4	n/a
Bolognese Sauce, cooked		145	8.0	3.7	11.1	1.1
	Dolmio	91.0	7.2	7.1	3.8	n/a
	Ragu	51.0	1.7	10.7	0.1	1.0
Bolognese Shells Italiana	Heinz Weight Watchers	71.0	5.2	9.6	1.3	0.8
Bombay Mix		503	18.8	35.1	32.9	6.2
	Holland & Barrett	524	16.4	38.4	33.9	6.2
	Sharwood	502	19.1	35.5	32.5	8.4
Bombay Potato Flat Bread, each	Boots Shapers	249	n/a	n/a	n/a	n/a
Bombay Spiced Poppadums	Sharwood	281	23.3	42.9	1.8	12.4
Boost	Cadbury	540	5.9	62.3	29.3	n/a
Boots Shapers Products: *see under individual products*						
Bounty, dark	Mars	481	3.2	57.4	26.5	n/a
milk	Mars	485	4.6	56.4	26.8	n/a
ice cream	Mars	331	4.2	28.2	22.4	n/a

All amounts given per 100g/100ml unless otherwise stated

Product	*Brand*	*Calories kcal*	*Protein (g)*	*Carbo-hydrate (g)*	*Fat (g)*	*Dietary Fibre (g)*
Bourbon Creams	Jacob's	477	5.7	69.6	19.6	1.7
Bournville	Cadbury	495	4.6	59.6	26.7	n/a
Bournvita Powder		341	7.7	79.0	1.5	N
made up with whole milk		76.0	3.4	7.6	3.8	Tr
made up with semi-skimmed milk		58.0	3.5	7.6	1.6	Tr
Boursin - Ail and Fines Herbs	Van den Bergh	414	7.0	2.0	42.0	Tr
au Poivre	Van den Bergh	414	7.0	2.0	42.0	Tr
au Naturel	Van den Bergh	423	7.0	2.0	43.0	n/a
Light	Van den Bergh	153	12.5	4.5	9.5	Tr
Bovril		169	38.0	2.9	0.7	nil
Bovril Beef Instant Drink	Bestfoods	194	43.6	3.8	0.5	2.0
Bovril Beef Stock Cubes	Bestfoods	173	9.1	24.8	4.1	Tr
Bovril Chicken Instant Drink	Bestfoods	140	10.9	22.2	0.8	n/a
Boysenberries in Syrup	Libby	68.0	n/a	n/a	Tr	n/a
Boysenberry Still Water	Boots Shapers	1.0	n/a	n/a	Tr	n/a

Braised Beef	Tyne Brand	102	10.9	3.2	5.1	n/a
Bramley Apple & Custard Pies	Mr Kipling	361	3.8	51.2	15.2	n/a
Bramley Apple Fruit Pie Bars	Mr Kipling	374	3.5	57.4	14.3	n/a
Bramley Apple Hot Cake	McVitie's	314	3.9	43.1	14.6	1.3
Bramley Apple Pies	Mr Kipling	345	3.4	53.6	12.6	n/a
individual	Mr Kipling	376	3.1	53.3	12.7	n/a
Bramley Apple Sauce	Colman's	108	0.2	26.0	Tr	n/a
Bran, wheat		206	14.1	26.8	5.5	39.6
Bran Cracker	Jacob's	456	9.5	63.2	18.3	2.9
Brandy: *see Spirits*						
Brandy Sauce Mix	Bird's	415	6.1	76.5	9.5	nil
Bran Fare	Weetabix	252	17.0	34.4	5.2	34.3
Bran Flakes	Kellogg's	320	10.0	66.0	2.0	15.0
Bran Oatcakes, each	Vessen	57.0	1.5	7.8	2.1	0.9

All amounts given per 100g/100ml unless otherwise stated

Product	*Brand*	*Calories kcal*	*Protein (g)*	*Carbo-hydrate (g)*	*Fat (g)*	*Dietary Fibre (g)*
Branston & Cheese French Bread Pizza	Findus	240	9.1	35.5	6.9	1.7
Branston Chilli	Crosse & Blackwell	130	0.7	30.0	0.1	1.5
Branston Original	Crosse & Blackwell	140	0.7	34.2	0.3	1.3
Branston Rich & Fruity	Crosse & Blackwell	110	0.5	24.3	0.1	1.1
Branston Sandwich Pickle	Crosse & Blackwell	140	0.7	34.2	0.3	1.3
Branston Tomato Pickle	Crosse & Blackwell	90.0	1.1	20.1	0.1	1.5
Brawn		153	12.4	nil	11.5	nil
Brazil Nuts		682	14.1	3.1	68.2	8.1
	Holland & Barrett	691	16.3	2.9	68.2	4.3

Bread (see also types)						
brown		218	8.5	44.3	2.0	5.9
	Heinz Weight Watchers	212	12.1	36.8	1.9	6.3
	Hovis	233	10.8	40.1	3.3	3.7
	Mothers Pride	218	8.1	42.8	1.5	4.6
	Sunblest	221	7.5	43.8	1.7	4.6
brown, toasted		272	10.4	56.5	2.1	7.1
currant		289	7.5	50.7	7.6	3.8
currant, toasted		323	8.4	56.8	8.5	4.2
French stick		270	9.6	55.4	2.7	5.1
granary		235	9.3	46.3	2.7	6.5
malt		268	8.3	56.8	2.4	6.5
pitta, white		265	9.2	57.9	1.2	3.9
rye		219	8.3	45.8	1.7	5.8
wheatgerm		212	9.5	41.5	2.0	5.1
wheatgerm, toasted		271	12.1	53.2	2.6	6.5
white		235	8.4	49.3	1.9	3.8
white, fried in oil/lard		503	7.9	48.5	32.2	3.8
white, toasted		265	9.3	57.1	1.6	4.5

All amounts given per 100g/100ml unless otherwise stated

Product	Brand	Calories kcal	Protein (g)	Carbo-hydrate (g)	Fat (g)	Dietary Fibre (g)
Bread (continued)						
wholemeal		215	9.2	41.6	2.5	7.4
wholemeal, toasted		252	10.8	48.7	2.9	8.7
Breaded Cod Fillets	Ross	180	11.1	17.9	7.4	0.8
Breaded Haddock Fillets	Ross	183	11.6	19.6	6.8	0.8
Breadfruit, canned, drained		66.0	0.6	16.4	0.2	2.5
Bread Pudding		297	5.9	49.7	9.6	3.0
Bread Rolls, brown, crusty		255	10.3	50.4	2.8	7.1
soft		268	10.0	51.8	3.8	6.4
Bread Rolls, white						
crusty		280	10.9	57.6	2.3	4.3
soft		268	9.2	51.6	4.2	3.9
Bread Rolls, wholemeal		241	9.0	48.3	2.9	8.8
Bread Sauce						
made with whole milk		150	4.1	10.9	10.3	0.6
made semi-skimmed milk		128	4.2	11.1	7.8	0.6

Bread Sauce Mix	Colman's	325	12.0	66.0	1.3	n/a
	Knorr	462	8.2	55.4	23.1	n/a
Breakfast Juice	Del Monte	43.0	0.6	9.6	Tr	n/a
Brie Cheese		319	19.3	Tr	26.9	nil
Broad Beans, boiled		48.0	5.1	5.6	0.8	5.4
frozen, boiled		81.0	7.9	11.7	0.6	6.5
canned		77.0	5.9	13.0	0.5	5.2
Broccoli, boiled		24.0	3.1	1.1	0.8	2.3
Broccoli & Cauliflower Cup-A-Soup Thick & Creamy, per sachet	Batchelors	120	1.9	17.2	4.8	0.6
Broccoli & Cauliflower Slim-A-Soup, per sachet	Batchelors	59.0	1.1	10.1	1.6	0.8
Broccoli & Potato Soup, organic	Baxters	31.0	1.3	5.8	0.3	0.7
Broccoli, Cauliflower & Potato Soup	Campbell's	34.0	0.6	5.0	1.3	n/a

All amounts given per 100g/100ml unless otherwise stated

Product	*Brand*	*Calories kcal*	*Protein (g)*	*Carbo-hydrate (g)*	*Fat (g)*	*Dietary Fibre (g)*
Broccoli Mix	Ross	41.0	2.3	9.0	0.5	2.3
Broccoli Soup	Baxters	41.0	1.1	5.0	1.9	0.4
Brown Ale, bottled		28.0	0.3	3.0	Tr	nil
Brown Bread: ***see Bread***						
Brown Lentils: ***see Lentils***						
Brown Rice: ***see Rice***						
Brown Ryvita, per slice	Ryvita	25.0	0.7	5.6	0.2	1.3
Brown Sauce, bottled		99.0	1.1	25.2	nil	0.7
	Burgess	102	0.8	22.0	0.2	1.1
	Daddies	102	0.9	24.3	0.6	n/a
Brussels Sprouts, boiled		35.0	2.9	3.5	1.3	2.6
Bubble & Squeak	Ross	111	1.7	13.8	6.0	1.3
Bulgur	Holland & Barrett	354	11.0	75.0	1.5	1.8
Buns: ***see individual flavours***						

Burgen Soya & Linseed Bread	Allied Bakeries	278	17.6	28.6	10.3	6.1
Burger Fun Pot Noodle	Golden Wonder	408	11.8	56.7	14.8	3.6
Burger Sauce	Burgess	594	2.2	10.7	59.9	nil
Butter		737	0.5	Tr	81.7	nil
	Kerrygold	720	n/a	Tr	80.0	nil
Butter Beans, dried, boiled		103	7.1	18.4	0.6	5.2
canned		77.0	5.9	13.0	0.5	4.6
	Batchelors	83.0	6.0	13.9	0.4	4.8
	Holland & Barrett	273	19.1	49.8	1.1	16.0
Buttermilk	Raines	40.0	4.3	5.5	0.1	n/a
Buttermint Bonbons	Cravens	425	0.5	86.1	8.7	nil
Butter Mintoes	Cravens	425	0.1	86.6	8.7	nil
Buttermints	Trebor Bassett	404	0.1	88.8	3.4	nil
Butterscotch	Cravens	411	0.1	89.9	5.7	nil
Buttons	Cadbury	525	7.8	56.8	29.4	n/a

All amounts given per 100g/100ml unless otherwise stated

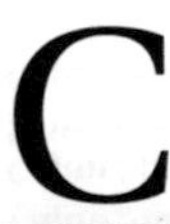

Product	Brand	Calories kcal	Protein (g)	Carbo-hydrate (g)	Fat (g)	Dietary Fibre (g)
Cabbage, average, raw		26.0	1.7	4.1	0.4	2.4
boiled		16.0	1.0	2.2	0.4	1.8
Cadbury's Caramel Dessert	St Ivel	210	3.5	31.6	7.7	nil
Cadbury's Crunchie Twinpot	St Ivel	248	5.1	29.8	12.0	nil
Cadbury's Flake Twinpot	St Ivel	257	5.6	27.4	13.9	nil
Cadbury's Milk Chocolate Dessert	St Ivel	260	4.8	20.5	17.6	nil
Cadbury's Milk Chocolate Mousse	St Ivel	166	5.3	22.8	5.9	nil

All amounts given per 100g/100ml unless otherwise stated

Product	*Brand*	*Calories kcal*	*Protein (g)*	*Carbo-hydrate (g)*	*Fat (g)*	*Dietary Fibre (g)*
Cadbury's Milk Chocolate Mousse (continued)						
low fat	St Ivel	123	4.9	15.3	4.7	nil
Cadbury's Milk Chocolate Trifle	St Ivel	278	5.1	24.2	17.9	Tr
Cadbury's Monty Mousse	St Ivel	166	5.3	22.8	5.9	nil
Caerphilly Cheese		375	23.2	0.1	31.3	nil
Caesar Style Low Fat Dressing	Heinz Weight Watchers	60.0	1.6	5.8	3.4	nil
Cajun Chicken Marinade	Birds Eye	172	15.2	8.7	8.5	0.9
Cajun 'Marinade in Minutes'	Knorr	254	4.0	55.6	1.7	n/a
Cajun Mustard	Colman's	187	7.0	23.0	6.5	2.7
Cajun Spicy Vegetable Slim-A-Soup, per sachet	Batchelors	57.0	1.6	10.4	1.0	1.2
Calabrese: ***see Broccoli***						

California Dreaming	Cadbury	480	6.7	59.6	23.9	n/a
Camembert		297	20.9	Tr	23.7	nil
Canada Dry Ginger Ale	Schweppes	37.5	Tr	9.1	nil	n/a
Cannelloni Bolognese	Dolmio	149	6.1	11.8	8.3	n/a
Cannelloni Cheese & Spinach Ready Meal	Dolmio	125	4.3	8.7	8.1	n/a
Cappuccino						
instant	Nescafé	386	10.6	62.8	10.3	nil
unsweetened	Nescafé	394	14.2	52.0	14.3	nil
Cappuccino Bar	Boots Shapers	346	n/a	n/a	13.0	n/a
Cappuccino Crunchy	Jordans	444	9.6	62.4	17.3	7.6
Capriccio, each	Nestlé	166	2.0	12.5	11.7	n/a
Captain's Cod Pie	Birds Eye	455	21.0	36.0	25.0	1.7
Caramac	Nestlé Rowntree	566	5.9	54.4	36.1	n/a
Caramac Breakaway	Nestlé Rowntree	526	6.3	56.0	30.7	n/a
Caramel	Cadbury	480	4.3	61.3	24.3	n/a

All amounts given per 100g/100ml unless otherwise stated

Product	*Brand*	*Calories kcal*	*Protein (g)*	*Carbo-hydrate (g)*	*Fat (g)*	*Dietary Fibre (g)*
Caramel & Walnut Cake	McVitie's	317	3.5	36.9	17.5	0.7
Caramel Bar	Boots Shapers	346	n/a	n/a	13.0	n/a
Caramel Cake Bars	Cadbury	410	5.9	56.1	16.8	n/a
Caramel Granymels	Itona	385	0.8	69.0	13.2	n/a
Caramel Harvest Chewy Bar, each	Quaker	93.0	1.3	14.3	3.3	0.7
Caramel Log	Tunnock's	472	4.2	64.3	24.0	n/a
Caramel Shortcake Bars	Mr Kipling	508	4.2	58.1	28.8	n/a
Caramel Shortcakes	Mr Kipling	482	3.8	54.7	27.5	n/a
Caramel Wafers	Tunnock's	454	4.6	68.0	20.1	n/a
Carbonara Creamy Pasta Bake	Napolina	101	3.8	9.6	5.3	0.1
Carbonara Pasta Choice	Crosse & Blackwell	380	14.9	58.3	9.7	2.6
Carbonara Pastaria Sauce	Knorr	511	8.9	44.1	33.2	0.2

Carbonara Pasta Sauce, chilled	Dolmio	180	3.6	4.6	16.4	n/a
jar	Dolmio	131	1.6	4.5	11.8	n/a
Carbonara Tastebreaks Pasta Snacks	Knorr	454	11.1	58.4	19.4	n/a
Caribbean Chicken Stir Fry	Ross	88.0	5.9	13.8	1.7	1.5
Caribbean Fruit Burst	Del Monte	39.0	0.1	9.5	Tr	n/a
Carmelle Mix	Green's	117	3.0	17.0	4.0	n/a
Carnation	Nestlé	160	8.2	11.5	9.0	nil
light	Nestlé	110	7.5	10.5	4.0	nil
Carrot & Butter Bean Soup	Baxters	47.0	1.6	6.8	1.7	2.3
Carrot & Coriander Soup	Baxters	38.0	0.8	5.5	1.4	0.8
Carrot & Lentil Soup	Heinz Weight Watchers	31.0	1.4	6.0	0.1	0.8
Carrot Cake	California Cake & Cookie Ltd	425	3.4	58.5	19.8	1.3

All amounts given per 100g/100ml unless otherwise stated

Product	Brand	Calories kcal	Protein (g)	Carbo-hydrate (g)	Fat (g)	Dietary Fibre (g)
Carrot Juice		24.0	0.5	5.7	0.1	N
Carrot, Onion & Chick Pea Soup	Baxters	34.0	1.7	7.1	0.1	1.5
Carrot, Potato & Coriander Soup	Heinz Weight Watchers	24.0	0.5	5.4	0.1	0.6
Carrots						
old, raw		35.0	0.6	7.9	0.3	2.4
old, boiled		24.0	0.6	4.9	0.4	2.5
young, raw		30.0	0.7	6.0	0.5	2.4
young, boiled		22.0	0.6	4.4	0.4	2.3
frozen, boiled		22.0	0.4	4.7	0.3	2.3
canned		20.0	0.5	4.2	0.3	1.9
Carrot with Parsnip and Nutmeg Soup, organic	Baxters	27.0	0.7	5.7	0.2	1.0
Cashew Nuts, roasted, salted		611	20.5	18.8	50.9	3.2
	Holland & Barrett	624	24.2	17.3	50.9	3.2

Cashew Pieces	Holland & Barrett	624	24.2	17.3	50.9	3.2
Cassava, fresh, raw		142	0.6	36.8	0.2	1.6
baked		155	0.7	40.1	0.2	1.7
boiled		130	0.5	33.5	0.2	1.4
Casserole Mix	Ross	22.0	0.9	6.2	0.2	1.8
Casserole Mixes (Colman's): ***see individual flavours***						
Caster Sugar	Tate & Lyle	400	nil	99.9	nil	nil
Cauliflower, raw		34.0	3.6	3.0	0.9	1.8
boiled		28.0	2.9	2.1	0.9	1.6
frozen, boiled		20.0	2.0	2.0	0.5	1.2
Cauliflower Cheese		105	5.9	5.1	6.9	1.3
	Birds Eye	108	4.8	7.7	6.4	0.8
Cauliflower CheeseJacket Potato	Birds Eye	97.0	3.2	14.1	3.1	1.1
Cauliflower Cheese Quarter Pounders, each	Birds Eye	220	7.0	17.0	14.0	2.1

All amounts given per 100g/100ml unless otherwise stated

Product	Brand	Calories kcal	Protein (g)	Carbo-hydrate (g)	Fat (g)	Dietary Fibre (g)
Cauliflower, Peas & Carrots	Birds Eye	32.0	2.2	4.8	0.4	2.6
Celeriac, raw		18.0	1.2	2.3	0.4	3.7
boiled		15.0	0.9	1.9	0.5	3.2
Celery, raw		7.0	0.5	0.9	0.2	1.1
boiled		8.0	0.5	0.8	0.3	3.2
Channa Masala	Sharwood	120	4.8	10.1	6.7	2.9
Chapati Flour, brown		333	11.5	73.7	1.2	N
white		335	9.8	77.6	0.5	N
Chapati, Paratha & Puri Mix	Sharwood	321	10.2	63.1	2.0	6.6
Chapatis, made with fat		328	8.1	48.3	12.8	N
made without fat		202	7.3	43.7	1.0	N
Chargrilled Chicken Salad Sandwich	Heinz Weight Watchers	153	9.4	17.7	4.9	2.1
Chasseur Cook-In-Sauce Classic	Homepride	45.0	0.8	9.2	0.4	n/a
Cheddar Cheese		412	25.5	0.1	34.4	nil

Cheddar Cheese Crispy Pancakes	Findus	185	6.4	23.5	7.5	0.8
Cheddar Cheese Dry Sauce Mix, per pack	Colman's	156	7.6	18.4	5.6	n/a
Cheddar Cheese Potato Bake Mix	Colman's	420	11.5	34.8	26.0	9.6
Cheddar Cheese & Onion Potato Bake Mix	Colman's	4.6	9.9	43.7	21.2	7.9
Cheddar Cheese Slices	Kraft	305	20.0	Tr	24.5	nil
Cheddar-type Cheese, reduced fat		261	31.5	Tr	15.0	nil
Cheddars	McVitie's	247	11.0	49.9	32.8	1.9
Cheese: *see individual types*						
Cheese & Bacon Pasta Bake	Homepride	104	2.4	2.6	9.3	n/a
Cheese & Bacon Pasta Bake Casserole Mix, per pack	Colman's	195	7.5	21.5	8.5	n/a
Cheese & Bacon Potato Bake	Homepride	215	1.8	0.6	22.9	n/a

All amounts given per 100g/100ml unless otherwise stated

Product	*Brand*	*Calories kcal*	*Protein (g)*	*Carbo-hydrate (g)*	*Fat (g)*	*Dietary Fibre (g)*
Cheese & Broccoli Chicken Lattice, each	Birds Eye	380	16.0	27.0	23.0	1.5
Cheese & Broccoli Pasta Bake	Birds Eye	132	12.5	6.1	6.4	0.3
Cheese & Broccoli with Tagliatelle Cup-A-Soup Extra, per sachet	Batchelors	160	5.2	23.5	5.0	1.9
Cheese & Chive Golden Lights, per pack	Golden Wonder	98.0	1.1	13.8	4.2	0.7
Cheese & Chives Soured Cream Dip	St Ivel	390	3.9	3.1	40.2	0.3
Cheese & Garlic Pasta 'n' Sauce	Batchelors	367	12.6	68.2	4.9	3.4
Cheese & Onion Crisps, per pack	Golden Wonder	131	1.5	12.3	8.4	1.2
Cheese & Onion Deep Topped Pizza Slices	McVitie's	223	8.4	30.3	8.2	1.3

Cheese & Onion Pizza, 5"	McCain	177	8.8	27.6	3.5	n/a
Cheese & Onion Potato Bake	Homepride	132	1.8	3.4	12.4	n/a
Cheese & Potato Bake	Tyne Brand	93.0	3.4	10.6	4.1	n/a
Cheese & Tomato Bronto's Monster Feet	McVitie's	240	10.2	33.0	8.1	1.3
Cheese & Tomato Crispy Pancakes	Findus					
Cheese & Tomato French Bread Pizza	Findus	235	9.3	32.4	7.8	1.8
Cheese & Tomato Pizza		235	9.0	24.8	11.8	1.5
	San Marco	244	11.8	24.7	11.3	1.0
5"	McCain	235	11.6	22.4	10.1	n/a
Cheeseburger, each	McDonald's	299	15.8	33.1	11.5	2.5
Cheesecake: *see also individual flavours*						
Cheesecake, frozen		242	5.7	33.0	10.6	0.9
Cheese, Leek & Ham Pasta 'n' Sauce	Batchelors	379	14.1	68.3	5.5	2.3

All amounts given per 100g/100ml unless otherwise stated

Product	Brand	Calories kcal	Protein (g)	Carbo-hydrate (g)	Fat (g)	Dietary Fibre (g)
Cheeselet	Jacob's	474	10.6	58.6	21.9	2.7
Cheese, Onion & Tomato Lasagne	Birds Eye	94.0	4.0	11.8	3.4	0.6
Cheese Ploughman's reduced fat cheese salad with pickle	Boots Shapers	330	21.0	39.0	10.0	6.6
Cheese Sauce						
made up with whole milk		197	8.0	9.0	14.6	0.2
with semi-skimmed milk		179	8.1	9.1	12.6	0.2
Cheese Sauce Packet Mix						
made up with whole milk		110	5.3	9.3	6.1	N
with semi-skimmed milk		90.0	5.4	9.5	3.8	N
	Knorr	495	8.4	35.9	35.1	0.1
Cheese Spread		276	13.5	4.4	22.8	nil
	Kerrygold	213	n/a	8.5	15.0	nil
per pack	Boots Shapers	86.0	n/a	n/a	3.1	n/a

Cheese Spread & Celery, per pack	Boots Shapers	88.0	n/a	n/a	3.1	n/a
Cheese Spread & Chives, per pack	Boots Shapers	87.0	n/a	n/a	3.1	n/a
Cheese Spread, Light	Primula	164	16.0	5.0	9.0	n/a
Cheese Spread, Original,	Primula	257	16.0	1.0	21.0	n/a
with Chives	Primula	253	15.0	1.0	21.0	n/a
with Ham	Primula	253	15.0	1.0	21.0	n/a
with Shrimp	Primula	253	15.0	1.0	21.0	n/a
with Sweet Pickle	Primula	273	13.0	8.0	21.0	n/a
with Tangy Tomato	Primula	257	15.0	2.0	21.0	n/a
with Tuna & Tomato	Primula	261	16.0	2.0	21.0	n/a
with Yeast Extract	Primula	257	16.0	1.0	21.0	n/a
Cheese, Tomato & Spring Onion with Mayonnaise Sandwiches, per pack	Boots Shapers	344	20.0	39.0	12.0	5.9
Cheese, Tomato & Vegetable Deep Crust Pizza Slice	McCain	193	9.4	26.7	5.4	n/a

All amounts given per 100g/100ml unless otherwise stated

Product	*Brand*	*Calories kcal*	*Protein (g)*	*Carbo-hydrate (g)*	*Fat (g)*	*Dietary Fibre (g)*
Cheese, Tomato & Vegetable Pizza Slice	McCain	159	7.4	27.8	2.8	n/a
Cheesey Croquette Royales	Ross	228	4.2	23.7	13.4	1.6
Cheesey Pasta, made up	Kraft	230	5.9	27.0	10.5	1.3
Cheesy Crackerbread	Ryvita	379	12.7	75.0	3.1	3.2
Cheesy Pasta Bake	Heinz Baked Bean Cuisine	106	5.0	14.3	3.2	1.4
Cheesy Wotsits, per pack	Golden Wonder	114	1.8	10.6	7.1	0.2
Chelsea Buns		366	7.8	56.1	13.8	1.7
Cherries, raw		48.0	0.9	11.5	0.1	0.9
canned in syrup		71.0	0.5	18.5	Tr	0.6
glacé		251	0.4	66.4	Tr	0.9
Cherryade	Corona	1.2	Tr	n/a	Tr	n/a
Cherry Bakewells	Mr Kipling	414	3.9	59.3	17.9	n/a
Cherry Bio Split Yogurt	Ski	124	4.5	8.3	4.0	nil

Cherry Brandy		255	Tr	32.6	nil	nil
Cherry Coke	Coca-Cola	45.0	nil	11.2	nil	n/a
Cherry Cream Cheesecake	McVitie's	336	4.9	30.0	22.0	1.4
Cherry Juice Special R, as sold	Robinsons	10.0	0.2	1.3	Tr	n/a
Cherry Pie Filling		82.0	0.4	21.5	Tr	0.4
Cherry Spring, per pack	Boots Shapers	3.0	n/a	n/a	Tr	n/a
Cheshire Cheese		379	24.0	0.1	31.4	nil
Chestnuts		170	2.0	36.6	2.7	4.1
Chewing Gum: ***see individual flavours***						
Chews (Trebor Bassett): ***see individual flavours***						
Chicken						
meat only, boiled		183	29.2	nil	7.3	nil
light meat, boiled		163	29.7	nil	4.9	nil
dark meat, boiled		204	28.6	nil	9.9	nil
meat only, roast		148	24.6	nil	5.4	nil
meat & skin, roasted		216	22.6	nil	14.0	nil

All amounts given per 100g/100ml unless otherwise stated

Product	*Brand*	*Calories kcal*	*Protein (g)*	*Carbo-hydrate (g)*	*Fat (g)*	*Dietary Fibre (g)*
Chicken (continued)						
light meat, roasted		142	26.5	nil	4.0	nil
dark meat, roasted		155	23.1	nil	6.9	nil
leg quarter, roast, meat only		92.0	15.4	nil	3.4	nil
wing quarter, roast, meat only		74.0	12.4	nil	2.7	nil
breaded, fried in veg. oil		242	18.0	14.8	12.7	0.7
Chicken à L'Orange	Findus Lean Cuisine	120	6.0	19.8	1.8	0.5
Chicken & Bacon Crispy Pancakes	Findus	165	6.4	23.3	4.9	0.9
Chicken & Bacon Lasagne	Findus Red Box	145	6.4	11.2	8.3	0.4
Chicken & Broccoli Pasta Bake	Heinz Weight Watchers	92.0	6.4	11.0	2.5	0.7
Chicken & Broccoli Pasta Snackpot, as sold	Findus Lean Cuisine	100	7.0	14.8	1.3	0.9

Chicken & Broccoli Soup	Knorr	313	8.8	54.2	6.8	2.4
Chicken & Ham Spread	Shippams	161	16.7	1.9	9.6	n/a
Chicken & Ham Soup	Heinz Big Soup	46.0	2.3	6.9	1.0	0.7
Chicken & Leek Cup Soup	Knorr	473	10.2	45.4	27.8	0.2
Chicken & Leek Soup	Campbell's	50.0	0.5	3.8	3.7	n/a
Chicken & Mayonnaise-Style Dressing Sandwich Filler	Heinz	191	6.3	7.7	15.0	0.3
Chicken & Mushroom Casserole, per pack	Birds Eye	165	18.0	5.0	8.0	0.6
Chicken & Mushroom Create-a-Stir	Findus	140	7.9	20.2	2.8	1.6
Chicken & Mushroom Crispy Pancake	Findus	165	5.7	23.4	5.5	0.9
Chicken & Mushroom Pasta 'n' Sauce	Batchelors	361	12.4	73.5	2.0	2.7
Chicken & Mushroom Pot Light	Golden Wonder	328	16.2	60.9	2.1	4.6

All amounts given per 100g/100ml unless otherwise stated

Product	*Brand*	*Calories kcal*	*Protein (g)*	*Carbo-hydrate (g)*	*Fat (g)*	*Dietary Fibre (g)*
Chicken & Mushroom Pot Meal, per pack	Boots Shapers	199	n/a	n/a	4.6	n/a
Chicken & Mushroom Pot Noodle	Golden Wonder	403	12.4	55.2	14.7	3.3
Chicken & Mushroom Potato Bake	Homepride	122	2.3	1.9	11.7	n/a
Chicken & Mushroom Slim-A-Soup, per sachet	Batchelors	59.0	1.4	8.4	2.2	0.6
Chicken & Mushroom Soup	Campbell's	43.0	0.5	3.5	3.1	n/a
Chicken & Mushroom Toast Toppers	Heinz	56.0	5.1	5.7	1.4	0.2
Chicken & Mushroom with Pasta Cup-A-Soup Extra, per sachet	Batchelors	144	4.0	21.8	4.5	1.5
Chicken & Prawn Creole Snackpot, as sold	Findus Lean Cuisine	100	5.2	14.9	1.9	0.8

Chicken & Sweetcorn Pasta Bake Casserole Mix, as sold	Colman's	329	12.0	58.0	5.2	n/a
Chicken & Sweetcorn Pot Rice	Golden Wonder	352	13.4	64.2	4.6	3.8
Chicken & Sweetcorn Slim-A-Soup, per sachet	Batchelors	59.0	1.2	9.2	1.9	0.3
Chicken & Sweetcorn Soup	Baxters	42.0	1.6	6.2	1.2	0.5
	Boots Shapers	40.0	n/a	n/a	1.2	n/a
Chicken & Vegetable Cup-A-Soup, per sachet	Batchelors	132	1.4	18.9	5.6	0.3
Chicken & Vegetable Pie	Ross	251	7.3	26.5	13.4	1.1
	Tyne Brand	162	4.7	14.3	9.6	n/a
Chicken & Vegetable Soup	Baxters	31.0	1.3	5.6	0.5	1.6
	Heinz Big Soups	47.0	2.4	7.3	1.0	0.9
Chicken & White Wine Soup	Campbell's	49.0	1.0	4.0	3.3	n/a
Chicken Biryani and Vegetable Rice, per pack	Birds Eye	430	14.0	48.0	20.0	4.3

All amounts given per 100g/100ml unless otherwise stated

Product	*Brand*	*Calories kcal*	*Protein (g)*	*Carbo-hydrate (g)*	*Fat (g)*	*Dietary Fibre (g)*
Chicken Breast in Gravy, per pack	Birds Eye	130	24.0	4.5	1.6	0.2
Chicken Broth	Baxters	34.0	1.2	5.3	0.9	0.6
Chicken Burgers, each	Birds Eye	150	7.8	9.6	8.7	0.2
Chicken Byriani Create-a Stir	Findus	110	5.0	18.0	2.5	2.1
Chicken Caesar Salad with Mixed Leaf Sandwiches, per pack	Boots Shapers	322	20.0	38.0	10.0	5.2
Chicken Casserole	Tyne Brand	100	4.2	7.1	6.3	n/a
Chicken Casserole & Dumplings	Shippams	130	9.5	9.4	6.0	n/a
Chicken Casserole & Mash, per pack	Birds Eye	350	19.0	32.0	16.0	2.5

Chicken Chasseur Casserole Mix, as sold	Colman's	273	12.0	53.0	1.0	n/a
Chicken Chasseur Classic Mix, as sold	Crosse & Blackwell	320	10.9	51.5	7.5	1.6
Chicken Cup-A-Soup, per sachet	Batchelors	98	1.5	12.4	4.7	0.6
Chicken Curry	Findus Red Box	125	6.0	18.1	3.1	0.8
	Tyne Brand	149	4.5	11.0	9.7	n/a
with rice	Heinz Weight Watchers	98.0	5.0	15.6	1.7	0.5
with rice, as sold	Vesta	376	13.4	64.1	7.4	3.6
with rice, per pack	Birds Eye	475	22.0	78.0	8.4	3.1
Chicken Curry Pot Rice	Golden Wonder	346	14.1	66.1	2.8	4.4
Chicken Curry with Chips, per meal	Birds Eye	420	18.0	46.0	18.0	5.4
Chicken Dhansak & Indian Potatoes	Findus Lean Cuisine	85.0	5.5	9.9	2.5	1.2

All amounts given per 100g/100ml unless otherwise stated

Product	*Brand*	*Calories kcal*	*Protein (g)*	*Carbo-hydrate (g)*	*Fat (g)*	*Dietary Fibre (g)*
Chicken Fahitas Mexican Creations Mix, as sold	Crosse & Blackwell	310	11.4	48.4	7.1	3.5
Chicken Granules, as sold	Oxo	296	11.1	52.4	4.9	0.7
Chicken Hotpot	Heinz Weight Watchers	89.0	5.0	11.4	2.6	0.9
Chicken in a Curry Dressing Sandwich Fillers	Shippams	167	7.5	11.7	10.0	n/a
Chicken in a Spicy Thai Dressing Sandwich Fillers	Shippams	139	7.4	8.7	8.3	n/a
Chicken in a Tikka Dressing Sandwich Fillers	Shippams	146	7.7	8.8	8.9	n/a
Chicken in Black Bean Sauce, per pack	Birds Eye	390	20.0	72.0	2.2	1.8
Chicken in Peppercorn Sauce	Heinz Weight Watchers	84.0	4.8	11.9	1.8	0.7

Chicken Jalfrezi Meal	Birds Eye	470	23.0	70.0	11.0	3.2
Chicken Kievs, each	Birds Eye	285	18.0	15.0	17.0	1.0
Chicken Korma Crispy Pancakes	Findus	170	6.9	22.8	5.9	1.0
Chicken Korma Readymeal	Uncle Ben's	123	9.1	6.3	6.8	n/a
Chicken Korma with Rice	Heinz Weight Watchers	97.0	5.8	13.5	2.1	0.2
Chicken McNuggets (6)	McDonald's	253	18.5	11.5	14.7	2.0
Chicken Mexicana with Rice	Heinz Weight Watchers	97.0	5.8	13.5	2.1	0.2
Chicken Micro Noodle	Knorr	477	8.4	57.0	24.0	n/a
Chicken Noodle Cup-A-Soup per sachet	Batchelors	89	3.7	15.9	1.2	0.5
Chicken Noodle Packet Soup	Batchelors	25	1.6	4.2	0.2	0.3
Chicken Noodle Soup, dried, as sold		329	13.8	60.9	5.0	4.3
dried, as served		20.0	0.8	3.7	0.3	0.2

All amounts given per 100g/100ml unless otherwise stated

Product	*Brand*	*Calories kcal*	*Protein (g)*	*Carbo-hydrate (g)*	*Fat (g)*	*Dietary Fibre (g)*
Chicken Noodle Soup	Heinz	27.0	1.1	4.9	0.3	0.2
	Heinz Weight Watchers	16.0	0.7	3.1	0.1	0.2
Chicken Oxo Cubes	Oxo	243	15.6	36.6	3.4	1.4
Chicken Pasta & Vegetable Soup	Heinz Big Soup	34.0	1.8	5.9	0.4	0.8
Chicken Quarter Pounder, each	Birds Eye	280	16.0	18.0	16.0	0.7
Chicken Ravioli in a Spicy Indian Sauce	Heinz	81.0	2.8	13.7	1.6	0.5
Chicken Rice Soup	Campbell's	26.0	0.7	4.5	0.7	n/a
Chicken Savoury Rice	Batchelors	357	9.9	74.5	2.2	2.9
Chicken Seasoning Dry Sauce Mix, as sold	Colman's	307	11.0	62.0	1.4	n/a
Chicken Soup	Heinz Weight Watchers	30.0	1.2	4.1	1.0	0.0

Chicken Spread	Shippams	151	18.5	1.9	7.7	n/a
Chicken Stew	Tyne Brand	74.0	2.8	5.9	4.4	n/a
Chicken Stew & Dumplings, per meal	Birds Eye	370	20.0	32.0	18.0	2.4
Chicken Stock Cubes	Knorr	301	10.1	23.6	18.5	0.2
Chicken Stock Powder	Knorr	163	12.2	18.0	4.7	0.2
Chicken Supernoodles	Batchelors	481	9.2	64.5	20.7	3.3
Chicken Supreme with rice	Heinz Weight Watchers	85.0	5.5	11.7	1.7	0.5
as sold	Vesta	401	15.3	59.9	11.2	3.0
per pack	Birds Eye	485	21.0	73.0	12.0	1.9
Chicken Supreme Casserole Mix, as sold	Colman's	399	16.0	48.0	15.0	n/a
Chicken Sweet & Sour Readymeal	Uncle Ben's	103	6.1	17.5	0.9	n/a
Chicken 3 Minute Noodles	Crosse & Blackwell	335	14.4	66.0	1.5	2.9

All amounts given per 100g/100ml unless otherwise stated

Product	*Brand*	*Calories kcal*	*Protein (g)*	*Carbo-hydrate (g)*	*Fat (g)*	*Dietary Fibre (g)*
Chicken Tikka & Mayonnaise Spread	Shippams	209	15.9	5.7	13.6	n/a
Chicken Tikka Chicken Tonight Sauce	Batchelors	130	2.2	9.6	9.2	1.7
Chicken Tikka Balti	Heinz Weight Watchers	71.0	4.2	10.	1.6	0.7
Chicken Tikka Masala Crisps, per pack	Golden Wonder	180	2.0	16.7	11.7	1.5
Chicken Tikka Masala Platter, per meal	Birds Eye	490	38.0	44.0	18.0	4.2
	Birds Eye Healthy Options	405	32.0	50.0	8.5	3.5
Chicken Tikka Sandwich	Heinz Weight Watchers	177	13.1	21.4	4.4	1.5
Chicken Tikka with Pilau Rice, per pack	Birds Eye	515	22.0	75.0	14.0	3.1

Chicken Tikka with Rice, as sold	Vesta	376	14.9	65.1	6.2	2.9
Chicken Tuscany & Pesto Tagliatelle, as sold	Findus Lean Cuisine	120	6.8	15.1	3.4	0.9
Chicken, Vegetable & Noodle Slim-A-Soup , per sachet	Batchelors	57.0	1.5	10.0	1.0	1.1
Chicken with Mild Korma Soup	Baxters	54.0	1.6	7.3	2.0	0.6
Chick Grills	Ross	324	9.9	21.3	22.5	0.9
Chick Peas						
dried, boiled		121	8.4	18.2	2.1	4.3
canned		115	7.2	16.1	2.9	4.1
Chick Pea Spread: *see Hummus*						
Chicksticks	Birds Eye	274	14.4	13.3	18.1	0.8
Chicory, raw		11.0	0.5	2.8	0.6	0.9
Chilli & Garlic Sauce	Amoy	112	12.0	27.0	n/a	n/a
	Lea & Perrins	60.0	1.0	14.9	Tr	n/a

All amounts given per 100g/100ml unless otherwise stated

Product	Brand	Calories kcal	Protein (g)	Carbo-hydrate (g)	Fat (g)	Dietary Fibre (g)
Chilli Beanfeast, per packet, as served	Batchelors	312	24.3	42.7	4.9	13.6
Chilli Bean Filler	Primula	203	6.4	12.0	15.0	2.7
Chilli Bean Spread, per pack	Boots Shapers	114	n/a	n/a	4.0	n/a
Chilli Beans		70.0	4.9	12.2	0.5	3.9
Chilli Beans in Sauce	Batchelors	101	8.3	16.0	0.4	3.8
Chilli Con Carne	Old El Paso	118	9.3	8.3	5.5	n/a
	Tyne Brand	106	9.4	6.6	4.7	n/a
per meal	Birds Eye	325	12.0	53.0	7.0	4.8
Chilli Con Carne Casserole Mix	Colman's	308	8.6	6.2	1.7	n/a
Chilli Con Carne Mexican Creations Mix, as sold	Crosse & Blackwell	320	14.0	32.3	14.6	8.8
Chilli Con Carne Sauce						
mild	Uncle Ben's	75.0	4.4	13.5	0.6	n/a
medium	Uncle Ben's	79.0	4.5	14.6	0.6	n/a

hot	Uncle Ben's	81.0	4.54	14.8	0.6	n/a
Chilli Cook-In-Sauce	Homepride	58.0	2.3	10.6	0.7	n/a
Chilli Mustard	Colman's	113	6.8	4.5	6.6	3.1
Chilli Peppers						
red, raw		26.0	1.8	4.2	0.3	N
green, raw		20.0	2.9	0.7	0.6	N
Chilli Sauce	HP	134	1.2	32.3	Tr	n/a
Chilli with Beans and Vegetables	Tyne Brand	111	5.9	12.5	4.2	n/a
China Fruit Salad in Syrup	Libby	70.0	n/a	n/a	Tr	n/a
Chinese Barbecue Cook-In-Sauce	Homepride	91.0	0.6	21.3	0.1	n/a
Chinese Chicken & Noodle Tastebreaks Soup	Knorr	419	11.8	66.5	11.8	n/a
Chinese Chicken & Prawn Foo Yeung Stir Fry	Ross	77.0	5.5	12.3	1.4	1.8

All amounts given per 100g/100ml unless otherwise stated

Product	*Brand*	*Calories kcal*	*Protein (g)*	*Carbo-hydrate (g)*	*Fat (g)*	*Dietary Fibre (g)*
Chinese Chicken Flavour Instant Noodles	Sharwood	483	10.2	56.0	17.7	2.3
Chinese Chicken Noodle Pot Light	Golden Wonder	329	14.1	62.7	2.4	5.5
Chinese Chicken Noodle Soup of the World	Knorr	337	15.6	57.0	5.2	n/a
Chinese Chicken Stir Fry	Ross	57.0	5.7	9.6	0.8	2.8
Chinese Chow Mein Supernoodles	Batchelors	481	9.7	63.5	20.8	3.0
Chinese Curry Flavour Instant Noodles	Sharwood	442	9.8	55.8	19.2	3.1
Chinese 'Marinades in Minutes'	Knorr	311	4.1	67.6	2.7	n/a
Chinese Mushroom, dried		284	10.0	59.9	1.8	Tr
Chinese Chicken Noodle Cup-A-Soup Extra, per sachet	Batchelors	101	3.5	19.1	1.2	2.0

Chinese Herb & Spice Cubes, each	Oxo	17.0	0.7	2.7	0.4	0.2
Chinese Pouring Sauces (Sharwood): ***see individual flavours***						
Chinese Prawns Stir Fry	Ross	60.0	3.3	12.4	0.4	1.5
Chinese Sauce Mixes (Sharwood): ***see individual flavours***						
Chinese Sizzling Prawns Stir Fry	Ross	39.0	3.3	8.2	0.3	2.5
Chinese Rices of the World	Batchelors	367	10.1	75.3	2.8	2.3
Chinese Special Rice	Ross	99.0	4.1	21.1	0.3	1.0
Chinese Spring Rolls	Ross	114	4.0	22.5	1.6	1.7
Chinese Sweet & Sour Make a Meal	Birds Eye	75.0	2.7	15.0	0.5	1.0
Chinese Sweet & Sour Pork Stir Fry	Ross	63.0	4.1	12.0	0.8	2.1
Chinese Szechuan Cooking Sauce	Heinz Weight Watchers	48.0	1.2	7.7	1.4	0.8

All amounts given per 100g/100ml unless otherwise stated

Product	Brand	Calories kcal	Protein (g)	Carbo-hydrate (g)	Fat (g)	Dietary Fibre (g)
Chinese Tomato & Noodle Soups of the World	Knorr	328	7.8	66.9	6.1	4.5
Chips						
crinkle cut, frozen, fried		290	3.6	33.4	16.7	2.2
French fries, retail		280	3.3	34.0	15.5	2.1
homemade, fried		189	3.9	30.1	6.7	2.2
retail		239	3.2	30.5	12.4	2.2
straight cut, frozen, fried		273	4.1	36.0	13.5	2.4
Chips, microwave		221	3.6	32.1	9.6	2.9
Chips, oven		162	3.2	29.8	4.2	2.0
Chip Shop Battered Fish Cakes	Ross	232	10.6	19.7	12.7	0.8
Chip Shop Chips	Ross	75.0	2.0	17.6	0.2	1.3
Chip Shop Fish Cakes	Ross	232	10.6	19.7	12.7	0.8
Chip Shop Jumbo Cod & Chips	Ross	169	6.1	19.1	7.9	0.8

Chip Shop Jumbo Cod Fish Fingers	Ross	232	10.2	14.2	15.2	0.7
Chip Shop Jumbo Cod Steaks	Ross	180	10.4	11.5	10.5	0.5
Chip Shop Jumbo Fish Steaks	Ross	186	11.0	13.9	9.9	0.6
Chip Shop Mushy Peas	Batchelors	78	4.9	13.8	0.3	3.3
	Ross	117	7.5	23.0	0.2	1.8
Chip Shop Scampi	Ross	228	8.3	22.8	11.9	1.0
Chip Shop Scampi Fries	Ross	228	8.3	22.8	11.9	0.9
Choc Chip & Hazelnut Cookies	McVitie's	504	5.4	65.2	24.3	2.0
Choc Chip & Orange Cookies	McVitie's	501	5.3	65.8	23.8	2.0
Choc Chip Harvest Chewy Bar, each	Quaker	94.0	1.3	14.1	3.5	0.7
Choc Chip Tracker	Mars	531	8.1	59.5	29.0	n/a
Chococino Hot Chcolate Drink, as sold	Nestlé	437	12.3	61.0	16.0	0.6

All amounts given per 100g/100ml unless otherwise stated

Product	Brand	Calories kcal	Protein (g)	Carbo-hydrate (g)	Fat (g)	Dietary Fibre (g)
Chococino Lite, as sold	Nestlé	345	15.8	51.0	8.6	3.8
Choco Corn Flakes	Kellogg's	380	6.0	84.0	2.5	2.5
Chocolate: *see individual flavours*						
Chocolate & Caramel Bar, per pack	Boots Shapers	97.0	n/a	n/a	4.9	n/a
Chocolate & Honeycomb Pieces Iced Dessert	Heinz Weight Watchers	159	3.1	26.2	4.3	0.8
Chocolate & Orange Royale	McVitie's	286	5.6	27.5	17.1	0.2
Chocolate Bar Cake	McVitie's	377	4.8	53.8	14.9	1.3
Chocolate Biscuits, full-coated		524	5.7	67.4	27.6	2.1
Chocolate Blancmange Powder, as sold	Brown & Polson	339	2.7	78.0	1.7	0.8
Chocolate Caramel Creams	Trebor Bassett	426	3.3	62.6	18.0	1.2
Chocolate Chip Cake Bars	Mr Kipling	457	5.5	45.3	25.9	n/a

Chocolate Chip Cookies	Cadbury	495	6.5	66.2	22.5	2.6
organic	Doves Farm	495	4.7	54.4	28.7	4.0
Chocolate Chip Solar	McVitie's	472	6.7	56.8	24.1	2.2
Chocolate Cream	Cadbury	425	2.6	68.8	15.4	n/a
Chocolate Creme de Creme, each	Lyons Maid	161	3.2	17.5	8.8	n/a
Chocolate Crusha	Burgess	175	nil	41.8	nil	nil
Chocolate Cup Cakes	Lyons Cakes	321	2.4	67.5	4.6	n/a
Chocolate Dessert	Chambourcy	220	4.4	25.4	11.3	1.0
Chocolate Dessert (in pots)	Provamel	93.0	3.0	14.9	2.3	1.3
Chocolate Digestive Bars	McVitie's	513	6.5	63.0	26.0	2.2
Chocolate Digestives: *see Digestive Biscuits*						
Chocolate Eclairs	Cravens	479	2.8	71.9	20.1	0.5
	Trebor Bassett	485	4.6	75.0	18.8	nil
Chocolate Farls	Tunnock's	521	5.5	62.8	27.5	n/a
Chocolate Flake Cake	Cadbury	417	6.0	48.0	21.1	n/a

All amounts given per 100g/100ml unless otherwise stated

Product	*Brand*	*Calories kcal*	*Protein (g)*	*Carbo-hydrate (g)*	*Fat (g)*	*Dietary Fibre (g)*
Chocolate Hob Nobs	McVitie's	497	6.3	62.8	24.3	3.7
Chocolate Homewheat	McVitie's	507	6.5	64.8	24.3	2.5
Chocolate Hot Crunch Pudding Mix	Bird's	445	6.3	72.5	14.0	1.0
Chocolate Ice Cream	Fiesta	187	3.5	20.6	10.6	n/a
	Lyons Maid	91.0	2.0	11.4	4.2	n/a
per pack	Boots Shapers	130	n/a	n/a	5.5	n/a
Chocolate Ice Dessert	Provamel	105	1.2	10.2	6.6	nil
Chocolate Jaspers	McVitie's	506	6.0	64.7	24.5	2.7
Chocolate Limes	Cravens	406	0.6	90.9	4.5	0.3
Chocolate M & Ms	Mars	487	4.7	69.6	21.1	n/a
Chocolate Mini Rolls	Cadbury	433	5.4	54.9	20.5	n/a
Chocolate Mint Crisp	Cravens	408	0.7	90.4	9.4	0.4
Chocolate Mousse		139	4.0	19.9	5.4	N

	Heinz Weight Watchers	97.0	4.8	10.3	3.6	0.4
each	Fiesta	83.0	1.9	10.2	3.8	n/a
Chocolate Nesquik	Nestlé	370	3.1	83.4	2.8	0.8
made up with whole milk	Nestlé	171	7.1	18.5	8.1	0.1
with semi-skimmed milk	Nestlé	155	7.3	22.8	3.7	0.1
ready to drink	Nestlé	68.0	3.4	11.6	1.7	0.2
Chocolate Nesquik Dessert	Nestlé	430	4.4	70.1	14.6	1.0
Chocolate Nut Spread		549	6.0	60.5	33.0	0.8
Chocolate Nut Sundae		278	3.0	34.2	15.3	0.1
Chocolate Oliver Biscuits	Fortts	359	6.5	69.5	23.9	3.9
Chocolate Orange Cake Bar	Jacob's Vitalinea	382	3.3	70.4	9.7	2.2
Chocolate Ready Brek	Weetabix	377	10.5	61.9	9.7	8.4
Chocolate Ripple Ice Cream	Lyons Maid	98.0	2.0	14.2	3.7	n/a
Chocolate Ripple Napoli	Lyons Maid	121	2.3	14.9	5.9	n/a
Chocolate Sandwich	Lyons Cakes	378	5.7	46.7	18.7	n/a

All amounts given per 100g/100ml unless otherwise stated

Product	*Brand*	*Calories kcal*	*Protein (g)*	*Carbo-hydrate (g)*	*Fat (g)*	*Dietary Fibre (g)*
Chocolate Snack Sandwich	Cadbury	525	7.2	62.6	27.2	n/a
Chocolate Squares	Mornflake	443	9.7	67.2	13.9	4.0
Chocolate Sundae, per pack	Boots Shapers	146	n/a	n/a	5.8	n/a
Chocolate Swirl Iced Dessert	Heinz Weight Watchers	133	2.6	19.6	4.6	0.5
Chocolate Swiss Roll	Lyons Cakes	384	5.4	50.8	15.8	n/a
Chocolate Tiramisu	Heinz Weight Watchers	181	4.1	26.9	3.7	0.8
Chocolate Trifle, per pack	Boots Shapers	117	n/a	n/a	4.9	n/a
Chocolate Truffle Cheesecake	McVitie's	340	5.9	35.4	19.7	0.6
Chocolate Truffles	Elizabeth Shaw					
Cointreau		475	3.8	63.2	22.3	0.3
Tia Maria		477	3.8	63.5	22.5	0.3
Irish Cream		477	3.9	63.4	22.8	0.3

Chocolate with Chocolate Sauce Sponge Pudding	Heinz	285	2.7	48.2	9.1	1.4
Chocolova	McVitie's	351	3.4	42.3	18.7	Tr
Chocomousse	Jacob's Vitalinea	366	3.7	67.8	8.9	0.8
Choice Grain Cracker	Jacob's	440	8.8	67.1	15.1	3.5
Choice Wholemeal Biscuits	McVitie's	481	7.6	66.5	19.9	6.5
Chomp	Cadbury	465	3.5	67.9	19.8	n/a
Chopped Ham & Pork, canned		275	14.4	1.4	23.6	0.3
Chopped Tomatoes	Napolina	15.0	1.2	2.5	Tr	n/a
for Bolognese	Napolina	24.0	1.4	5.0	Tr	n/a
with Herbs	Napolina	15.0	1.2	2.5	Tr	n/a
with Onions & Herbs	Napolina	16.0	1.2	3.0	Tr	n/a
Chop Suey Stir Fry Sauce	Sharwood	75.0	0.7	14.6	1.5	0.2
Chow Mein, as sold	Vesta	318	14.8	54.0	4.7	7.7
Chow Mein Mix	Ross	58.0	2.2	13.3	0.4	1.8
Chow Mein Pot Noodle	Golden Wonder	424	12.9	59.3	15.0	3.2

All amounts given per 100g/100ml unless otherwise stated

Product	Brand	Calories kcal	Protein (g)	Carbo-hydrate (g)	Fat (g)	Dietary Fibre (g)
Christmas Pudding, recipe		291	4.6	49.5	9.7	1.3
retail		329	3.0	56.3	11.8	1.7
Christmas Slices	Mr Kipling	338	2.5	63.8	7.3	n/a
Chunky Chicken Supreme	Shippams	174	12.5	4.0	12.0	n/a
Chunky Chips	Ross	118	2.4	21.9	3.0	1.6
Chunky Onions and Garlic Sauce	Ragu	58.0	2.3	9.2	1.3	n/a
Chunky Sweet Pepper Sauce	Ragu	54.0	1.7	6.0	2.6	2.3
Chunky Vegetable Sauce	Ragu	59.0	2.0	7.0	2.6	2.5
Chutney: *see individual flavours*						
Cider, dry		36.0	Tr	2.6	nil	nil
sweet		42.0	Tr	4.3	nil	nil
vintage		101	Tr	7.3	nil	nil
low alcohol	Strongbow	16.0	n/a	n/a	n/a	n/a

Cinnamon Toast Crunch	Nestlé	416	4.6	75.1	10.9	4.2
Citrus Fruit Drink, per pack	Boots Shapers	nil	n/a	n/a	nil	n/a
Citrus Promise Dessert	St Ivel Shape	100	2.0	20.0	1.3	1.3
Classic Barbecue Sauce	HP	145	0.4	34.5	Tr	n/a
Classic Bean Salad	Batchelors	98.0	5.7	19.8	1.1	3.6
Classic Chinese Marinade	Sharwood	115	1.8	16.1	4.8	1.0
Clementines, flesh only		37	0.9	8.7	0.1	1.2
Clementines in Natural Juice	Libby	41.0	n/a	n/a	Tr	n/a
Cloudy Lemonade	Boots Shapers	2.0	n/a	n/a	Tr	n/a
Clover	Dairy Crest	682	n/a	n/a	75.0	n/a
Club Biscuits (Jacob's): *see individual flavours*						
Clusters	Nestlé	386	10.6	68.1	8.0	8.4
Coca-Cola		39.0	Tr	10.5	nil	nil
	Coca-Cola	43.0	nil	10.6	nil	n/a
Cock-a-Leekie Soup	Baxters	29.0	0.9	4.0	1.0	0.3

All amounts given per 100g/100ml unless otherwise stated

Product	Brand	Calories kcal	Protein (g)	Carbo-hydrate (g)	Fat (g)	Dietary Fibre (g)
Cockles, boiled		48.0	17.2	Tr	2.0	nil
Cocktail Cherries	Burgess	247	0.3	61.4	nil	10.0
Cocktail Dressing, low fat	Crosse & Blackwell	145	1.0	14.4	8.9	0.3
Cocoa Powder		312	18.5	11.5	21.7	12.1
made up with whole milk		76.0	3.4	6.8	4.2	0.2
made up with semi-skimmed milk		57.0	3.5	7.0	1.9	0.2
organic	Green & Black's	322	23.0	10.5	21.0	nil
Coconut, creamed		669	6.0	7.0	68.8	N
desiccated		604	5.6	6.4	62.0	13.7
Coconut & Pineapple Yogurt Mousse, per pack	Boots Shapers	80.0	n/a	n/a	3.7	n/a
Coconut Bar	Boots Shapers	346	n/a	n/a	13.0	n/a
Coconut Hot Chocolate, per pack	Boots Shapers	40.0	n/a	n/a	0.9	n/a
Coconut Oil		899	Tr	nil	99.9	nil

Coconut Sandwich	Lyons Cakes	391	4.2	50.7	18.1	n/a
Coco Pops	Kellogg's	380	4.5	85.0	2.0	2.5
Cod, dried, salted, boiled		138	32.5	nil	0.9	nil
Cod & Prawn Pie	Ross	164	8.7	11.9	9.3	0.5
Cod Crumble	Ross	179	8.9	12.7	10.5	0.5
Cod Fillet Fish Cakes in Crispy Crunch Crumb, each	Birds Eye Captain's Table	85.0	4.5	8.5	3.5	0.3
Cod Fillet Fish Fingers	Ross	182	11.5	17.4	8.7	0.7
	Birds Eye	177	12.7	14.1	7.7	1.0
Cod Fillets						
baked		96.0	21.4	nil	1.2	nil
poached		94.0	20.9	nil	1.1	nil
in Natural Crumb	Ross	180	11.1	17.9	7.4	0.8
Cod Fish Fingers	Ross	182	11.5	17.4	8.7	0.7
Cod Liver Oil		899	Tr	nil	99.9	nil
Cod Roe, hard, fried		202	20.9	3.0	11.9	0.1

All amounts given per 100g/100ml unless otherwise stated

Product	Brand	Calories kcal	Protein (g)	Carbo-hydrate (g)	Fat (g)	Dietary Fibre (g)
Cod Steak in Butter Sauce	Ross	84.0	10.5	3.0	3.4	0.1
	Birds Eye	97.0	10.0	3.9	4.6	0.1
Cod Steak in Cheese Sauce	Birds Eye	96.0	10.9	5.2	3.5	0.1
Cod Steak in Mushroom Sauce	Birds Eye	99.0	9.8	5.0	4.4	0.1
Cod Steak in Parsley Sauce	Ross	89.0	10.4	2.9	4.0	0.1
	Birds Eye	85.0	10.4	5.0	2.6	0.1
Cod Steaks						
grilled		95.0	20.8	nil	1.3	nil
in batter, fried in oil		199	19.6	nil	10.3	0.3
	Birds Eye	70.0	17.0	nil	0.3	nil
Cod Steaks in Crispy Crunch Crumb, each	Birds Eye	225	14.0	13.0	13.0	0.9
Cod Steaks in Natural Crumb	Ross	180	11.1	17.9	7.4	0.8
Coffee, infusion, 5 minutes		2.0	0.2	0.3	Tr	nil
instant		100	14.6	11.0	Tr	nil

Coffeemate, per 6.5g tsp						
regular	Carnation	35.0	Tr	3.9	2.0	nil
lite	Carnation	30.0	Tr	5.1	0.8	nil
Coffee Napoli	Lyons Maid	98.0	1.9	10.4	5.5	n/a
Coleslaw	Heinz	135	1.6	9.4	10.2	1.2
Coley Fillet, steamed		99.0	23.3	nil	0.6	nil
Common Sense Oat Bran Flakes	Kellogg's	340	11.0	64.0	5.0	11.0
Complete Custard Mix	Rowntree	412	4.2	77.8	10.2	n/a
Compound Cooking Fat		894	Tr	Tr	99.3	nil
Condensed Milk						
sweetened, skimmed		267	10.0	60.0	0.2	nil
sweetened, whole		333	8.5	55.5	10.1	nil
Conservation Grade Porridge Oats	Jordans	363	12.5	61.5	7.4	8.0
Consomme	Campbell's	7.0	1.3	0.5	nil	n/a
Continental Mix	Ross	37.0	1.6	8.9	0.4	2.2

All amounts given per 100g/100ml unless otherwise stated

Product	Brand	Calories kcal	Protein (g)	Carbo-hydrate (g)	Fat (g)	Dietary Fibre (g)
Cookeen Cooking fat	Van den Bergh	900	nil	nil	100	nil
Cooking Mixes and Sauces (Colman's): ***see individual flavours***						
Coolmints	Trebor Bassett	237	nil	98.7	nil	nil
Coq au Vin Casserole Mix, as sold	Colman's	281	7.5	59.0	1.0	n/a
Coriander & Herbs Delicately Flavoured Rice	Batchelors	369	7.9	79.6	3.5	5.0
Corned Beef, canned		217	26.9	nil	26.9	nil
	Libby	224	24.5	1.0	13.5	nil
Corn Flakes	Kellogg's	370	8.0	82.0	0.8	3.0
organic	Doves Farm	362	7.0	81.1	0.7	4.5
Cornflour		354	0.6	92.0	0.7	0.1
Cornish Ice Cream	Lyons Maid	92.0	19.	11.3	4.4	n/a
Cornish Pastie		332	8.0	31.1	20.4	0.9
Cornish Wafers	Jacob's	528	8.3	53.7	31.1	2.3

Corn Oil	Mazola	900	Tr	nil	100	nil
Corn on the Cob, whole, raw		54.0	2.0	9.9	1.0	0.9
boiled		66.0	2.5	11.6	1.4	1.3
Corn Pops	Kellogg's	380	6.0	85.0	2.0	2.0
Coronation Chicken with Mixed Leaf and Mayonnaise Sandwich	Boots Shapers	337	16.0	39.0	13.0	5.1
Coronation Sauce	Heinz	334	0.8	13.1	31.0	0.9
Cottage Cheese						
plain		98.0	13.8	2.1	3.9	nil
	St Ivel Shape	67.0	10.8	5.5	0.2	nil
with additions		95.0	12.8	2.6	3.8	Tr
with Nectarine & Apricot	St Ivel Shape	75.0	10.6	6.9	0.3	Tr
reduced fat		78.0	13.3	3.3	1.4	Tr
Cherry Tomato & Basil	St. Ivel Shape	73.0	10.9	4.5	1.0	0.1
Thai Style Prawn	St Ivel Shape	79.0	11.8	4.2	1.4	nil
Cough Candy	Cravens	386	Tr	96.4	nil	nil
	Trebor Bassett	383	nil	95.0	nil	nil

All amounts given per 100g/100ml unless otherwise stated

Product	Brand	Calories kcal	Protein (g)	Carbo-hydrate (g)	Fat (g)	Dietary Fibre (g)
Country Choice Harvester Rolls, each	Allied Bakeries	148	6.4	28.5	0.9	2.1
Country French Chicken Tonight Sauce	Batchelors	98.0	0.7	3.3	9.1	0.7
Country Garden Soup	Baxters	28.0	0.7	5.4	0.5	0.8
Country Grain Wholemeal Bread	Hovis	222	11.2	37.4	3.1	5.7
Country Mix Vegetables	Ross	31.0	2.1	6.8	0.5	2.4
Country Pork Casserole Classic Creations Mix, as sold	Crosse & Blackwell	350	6.1	62.8	7.3	1.7
Country Slices	Mr Kipling	380	4.8	56.2	15.1	n/a
Country Store	Kellogg's	360	9.0	69.0	5.0	7.0
Country Tomato & Bean Wholesoup, as served	Batchelors	325	15.8	68.0	3.5	10.3
Country Tomato Reduced Calorie Soup	Batchelors	27.0	1.6	4.1	0.4	n/a

Country Tomato Soup	Batchelors	60.0	1.4	6.3	3.3	n/a
Country Vegetable Soup	Heinz	51.0	2.3	9.3	0.5	1.1
	Heinz Weight Watchers	30.0	1.1	5.8	0.2	1.0
Courgettes (zucchini, squash), raw		18.0	1.8	1.8	0.4	0.9
boiled		19.0	2.0	2.0	0.4	1.2
fried in corn oil		63.0	2.6	2.6	4.8	1.2
Coucous	Holland & Barrett	355	13.5	72.5	1.9	2.0
Crab, boiled		127	20.1	nil	5.2	nil
canned		81.0	18.1	nil	0.9	nil
Crab Spread	Shippams	161	15.5	4.7	8.9	n/a
Cracker Barrel Cheddar Cheese	Kraft	410	26.0	0.1	34.0	nil
Crackerbread	Ryvita	383	9.8	79.3	3.0	2.6
with high fibre	Ryvita	318	12.6	60.5	2.8	16.8
Cranberry & Orange Sauce	Colman's	274	0.2	67.0	0.2	n/a
Cranberry Jelly	Baxters	268	nil	67.0	nil	nil

All amounts given per 100g/100ml unless otherwise stated

Product	*Brand*	*Calories kcal*	*Protein (g)*	*Carbo-hydrate (g)*	*Fat (g)*	*Dietary Fibre (g)*
Cranberry Sauce	Baxters	126	0.1	33.3	nil	1.4
	Burgess	180	0.1	45.0	nil	0.5
Cream, fresh (pasteurised)						
clotted		586	1.6	2.3	63.5	nil
double		449	1.7	2.7	48.0	nil
half		148	3.0	4.3	13.3	nil
single		198	2.6	4.1	19.1	nil
soured		205	2.9	3.8	19.9	nil
whipping		373	2.0	3.1	39.3	nil
Cream, sterilised, canned		239	2.5	3.7	23.9	nil
Cream, UHT, aerosol spray		309	1.9	3.5	32.0	nil
Cream Cheese		439	3.1	Tr	47.4	nil
Cream Cheese & Broccoli Potato Bake Mix	Colman's	410	7.4	43.2	23.1	8.4
Cream Crackers		440	9.5	68.3	16.3	2.2
	Jacob's	439	9.9	67.1	14.5	2.9
	Jacob's Vitalinea	397	10.2	71.7	7.7	3.1

Creamed Garlic Sauce	Burgess	424	2.5	20.9	36.1	1.6
Creamed Horseradish	Burgess	184	2.4	19.6	9.8	2.3
	Colman's	229	4.3	21.4	13.3	n/a
Creamed Macaroni	Ambrosia	88.0	3.6	14.6	1.7	0.3
Creamed Rice	Ambrosia	90.0	3.1	15.2	1.9	Tr
low fat	Ambrosia	81.0	3.2	15.2	0.8	Tr
Creamed Rice Pudding	Fussell's	89.0	3.1	15.4	1.6	0.2
	Libby	89.0	3.1	15.4	1.6	0.2
Creamed Rice Pudding Dessert Pots	Ambrosia	101	3.2	16.5	2.5	Tr
Creamed Sago	Ambrosia	79.0	2.5	13.6	1.6	nil
Creamed Semolina	Ambrosia	81.0	3.3	13.1	1.7	0.2
Creamed Tapioca	Ambrosia	80.0	2.5	13.8	1.6	nil
Cream 'n' Cheesy Nik Naks, per pack	Golden Wonder	186	1.7	19.1	11.4	0.4
Cream of Asparagus Soup	Baxters	64.0	1.2	5.3	4.2	0.2
	Campbell's	45.0	0.5	4.6	2.8	n/a
	Heinz	46.0	1.1	4.5	2.6	0.2

All amounts given per 100g/100ml unless otherwise stated

Product	Brand	Calories kcal	Protein (g)	Carbo-hydrate (g)	Fat (g)	Dietary Fibre (g)
Cream of Asparagus Real Soup in Seconds	Knorr	551	7.2	42.8	35.4	1.0
Cream of Cauliflower & Broccoli	Knorr	507	7.0	46.0	32.8	0.7
Cream of Celery Soup	Campbell's	47.0	0.6	3.2	3.4	n/a
	Heinz	44.0	0.8	4.1	2.7	0.2
Cream of Chicken & Mushroom Soup	Heinz	50.0	1.3	4.6	2.9	0.1
Cream of Chicken & Mushroom Soup	Knorr	520	7.7	42.8	35.4	0.8
Cream of Chicken Packet Soup	Batchelors	57.0	1.1	5.6	3.3	0.3
Cream of Chicken Soup,						
canned, ready to serve		58.0	1.7	4.5	3.8	N
condensed, ready to serve		98.0	2.6	6.0	7.2	N
	Campbell's	50.0	1.0	3.7	3.5	n/a
	Heinz	52.0	1.3	4.4	3.2	0.1

	Knorr	355	9.8	54.8	10.7	0.5
Cream of Garden Vegetable Packet Soup	Batchelors	51	1.2	6.6	2.2	0.6
Cream of Leek Real Soup in Seconds	Knorr	508	5.9	45.3	33.6	1.3
Cream of Leek Soup	Baxters	46.0	0.7	5.2	2.5	0.4
Cream of Mushroom Packet Soup	Batchelors	58.0	0.7	6.5	3.1	0.1
Cream of Mushroom Soup, canned, ready to serve		53	1.1	3.9	3.8	N
	Campbell's	52.0	0.6	3.6	3.9	n/a
	Knorr	437	9.7	47.8	23.0	n/a
Cream of Mushroom Real Soup in Seconds	Knorr	522	5.1	44.9	35.8	1.0
Cream of Onion Soup	Campbell's	42.0	0.5	3.7	2.9	n/a
Cream of Tomato Soup canned, ready to serve		55.0	0.8	5.9	3.3	N
	Baxters	71.0	1.5	10.6	2.5	0.7

All amounts given per 100g/100ml unless otherwise stated

Product	Brand	Calories kcal	Protein (g)	Carbo-hydrate (g)	Fat (g)	Dietary Fibre (g)
Cream of Tomato Soup (continued)						
	Heinz	64.0	0.9	7.1	3.6	0.4
condensed, ready to serve		123	1.7	14.6	6.8	N
	Campbell's	66.0	0.7	7.6	3.6	n/a
	Knorr	426	3.5	54.2	21.7	2.5
Cream of Vegetable Cup-A-Soup, per sachet	Batchelors	134	1.9	19.7	5.3	2.0
Cream Soda	Barr	29.0	Tr	7.2	Tr	Tr
	Idris	22.0	nil	5.3	nil	n/a
Cream Toffees, Assorted	Trebor Bassett	433	3.7	73.3	13.8	nil
Creamy Banana Oatso Simple	Quaker	372	7.5	72.0	5.5	4.5
Creamy Chardonnay Wine Pour Over Sauce	Baxters	98.0	1.5	6.6	7.4	0.1
Creamy Cheese Pasta Snack Stop	Crosse & Blackwell	123	4.0	16.6	4.5	n/a

Creamy Chicken & Sweetcorn Tastebreaks Soup	Knorr	519	11.3	50.5	3.02	n/a
Creamy Chicken Snack Stop	Crosse & Blackwell	99	2.7	15.0	3.2	n/a
Creamy Chicken Curry	Colman's	371	11.0	49.0	14.0	n/a
Creamy Curry Chicken Tonight Sauce	Batchelors	85	1.5	4.6	6.7	0.8
Creamy Curry Low In Fat Sauce	Homepride	54.0	1.4	9.2	1.5	n/a
Creamy Four Cheese Pour Over Sauce	Baxters	104	4.0	5.2	7.4	0.1
Creamy Garlic Sauce	Knorr	361	14.2	49.7	11.7	0.2
Creamy Hollandaise Sauce	Knorr	354	12.1	55.6	9.2	0.8
Creamy Mushroom &Garlic Cook-In-Sauce	Homepride	76.0	0.8	5.0	5.9	n/a
Creamy Mushroom Chicken Lattice, each	Birds Eye	415	16.0	31.0	25.0	1.7

All amounts given per 100g/100ml unless otherwise stated

Product	*Brand*	*Calories kcal*	*Protein (g)*	*Carbo-hydrate (g)*	*Fat (g)*	*Dietary Fibre (g)*
Creamy Mushroom Chicken Tonight Sauce	Batchelors	88.0	0.7	2.8	8.2	0.4
Creamy Mushgroom Pasta Bake	Homepride	112	1.8	2.9	10.3	n/a
Creamy Mushroom Pour over Sauce	Baxters	92.0	1.3	6.3	6.8	0.2
Creamy Mushroom Sauce	Knorr	341	12.7	49.7	10.1	1.7
Creamy Pepper Sauce	Knorr	332	11.3	51.1	9.1	3.0
Creamy Peppered Pork Dry Mix, as sold	Crosse & Blackwell	375	8.5	50.4	15.3	1.8
Creamy Pesto Pastaria Sauce	Knorr	490	8.8	43.2	31.3	0.5
Creamy Potato & Leek Tastebreaks Soup	Knorr	510	7.9	54.6	28.9	n/a
Creamy Rice with Strawberry Crunch	Ambrosia	144	3.9	23.0	4.2	0.7

Creamy Rice with Tropical Crunch	Ambrosia	144	3.6	23.2	4.2	0.7
Creamy Tomato & Herb Pasta Bakes	Homepride	99.0	1.7	7.2	7.0	n/a
Creamy Tomato & Mushroom Pasta 'n' Sauce, as served	Batchelors	366	13.0	71.0	3.3	3.2
Creamy Tomato &Pesto Premium Pasta Sauce	Napolina	87.0	2.2	9.3	4.6	0.8
Creamy Vegetable Tastebreaks Pasta Snacks	Knorr	432	10.3	60.7	16.4	n/a
Creme Caramel		109	3.0	20.6	2.2	N
	Chambourcy La Laitiere	115	4.9	20.4	1.6	nil
Creme Eggs		385	4.1	58.0	16.8	Tr
Creole Chicken Deep South Recipe	Homepride	78.0	1.5	13.7	2.1	n/a
Crinkle Cut Chips	McCain	139	2.4	21.7	4.7	n/a
Crinkle Cut Oven Chips	McCain	157	1.9	26.7	4.7	n/a

All amounts given per 100g/100ml unless otherwise stated

Product	*Brand*	*Calories kcal*	*Protein (g)*	*Carbo-hydrate (g)*	*Fat (g)*	*Dietary Fibre (g)*
Crisps: ***see individual flavours***						
Crispy Bacon Wheat Crunchies	Golden Wonder	172	3.9	19.6	8.7	1.0
Crispy Caramel Bar	Boots Shapers	376	n/a	n/a	17.0	n/a
Crispy Chicken and Chips, per meal	Birds Eye	510	22.0	54.0	23.0	4.8
Crispy Chinese Mix	Ross	36.0	2.0	6.9	0.4	1.0
Crispy Fish Dip-Ins	Birds Eye	229	10.7	15.6	13.7	0.7
Crispy Muesli	Jordans	416	10.1	66.0	9.3	6.9
Crispy Potato Fritters	Birds Eye	174	2.2	17.2	10.7	1.3
Crispy Vegetable Fingers	Birds Eye	171	3.8	21.0	8.0	1.2
Crofters' Thick Vegetable Soup	Knorr	300	10.7	56.9	3.3	4.8
Croissants		360	8.3	38.3	20.3	2.5
	International Harvest	459	8.5	36.9	30.8	1.2

Croquette Potatoes, each	Birds Eye	45.0	1.0	6.5	1.5	0.3
Crumble Mix	Whitworths	422	5.5	67.6	16.3	1.5
Crumpets, each	Sunblest	86.0	2.6	18.8	0.4	0.8
Crunchie	Cadbury	470	4.4	72.1	18.1	n/a
Crunchy Cereal, per 40g serving with skimmed milk	Boots Shapers	180	n/a	n/a	5.2	n/a
Crunchy Garlic Chicken	Birds Eye	262	14.4	16.9	15.2	0.9
Crunchy Nut Chex	Weetabix	384	6.5	80.9	3.8	3.7
Crunchy Nut Cornflakes	Kellogg's	390	7.0	82.0	3.5	2.5
Crunchy Peanut Butter	Holland & Barrett	591	25.5	10.3	49.8	7.4
	Sunpat	620	25.8	14.5	50.9	6.5
Crusha (Burgess): ***see individual flavours***						
Cube Sugar, white	Tate & Lyle	400	nil	99.9	nil	nil
Cucumber, raw		10.0	0.7	1.5	0.1	0.6

Product	Brand	Calories kcal	Protein (g)	Carbo-hydrate (g)	Fat (g)	Dietary Fibre (g)
Cucumber Sandwich Spread	Heinz	185	1.3	18.9	11.5	0.5
Cullen Skink Soup	Baxters	85.0	6.6	7.9	3.2	0.5
Cultured Buttermilk	Raines	40.0	4.3	5.5	0.1	nil
Curacao		311	Tr	28.3	nil	nil
Curly Kale, raw		33.0	3.4	1.4	1.6	3.1
boiled		24.0	2.4	1.0	1.1	2.8
Curly Wurly	Cadbury	450	4.8	69.9	16.7	n/a
Currant Buns		296	7.6	52.7	7.5	N
	Sunblest	298	7.2	52.6	6.5	2.0
Currant Crunch Ryvita, per slice	Ryvita	48.0	1.3	10.1	0.3	1.9
Currants, dried		267	2.3	67.8	0.4	1.9
	Holland & Barrett	248	2.3	67.7	0.4	1.9

Curried Baked Beans	Heinz	103	4.9	17.9	1.3	4.0
Curried Beef & Vegetables	Tyne Brand	87.0	3.7	11.0	3.4	n/a
Curried Chicken Sandwich Filler	Heinz	192	6.2	9.6	14.2	0.7
Curried Fruit Chutney	Sharwood	129	1.0	30.3	0.4	2.6
Curried Mince & Vegetables	Tyne Brand	100	5.7	9.6	4.3	n/a
Curry & Mango Dip	Primula	334	4.5	6.1	32.4	n/a
Curry Cook-In-Sauce	Homepride	105	0.9	8.9	7.2	n/a
Curry Sauce	HP	124	1.4	26.3	2.4	n/a
Curry Sauce, canned		78.0	1.5	7.1	5.0	N
Curry Sauce Dry Mix, as sold	Colman's	368	7.5	65.0	8.4	n/a
Curry 3 Minute Noodles	Crosse & Blackwell	340	14.4	65.0	2.4	3.1
Custard ***made up with whole milk***		117	3.7	16.6	4.5	Tr

All amounts given per 100g/100ml unless otherwise stated

Product	Brand	Calories kcal	Protein (g)	Carbo-hydrate (g)	Fat (g)	Dietary Fibre (g)
Custard (continued)						
made up with skimmed milk		79.0	3.8	16.8	0.1	Tr
canned		95.0	2.6	15.4	3.0	0.1
canned, low fat	Ambrosia	72.0	2.9	12.7	1.1	0.1
powder	Creamola	350	0.4	92.0	0.7	n/a
	Bird's	355	0.4	87.0	0.5	nil
ready to serve	Bird's	102	2.8	15.5	3.0	nil
Custard Creams	Jacob's	482	5.4	68.3	20.7	1.6
each	Crawford's	62.0	0.8	8.2	2.9	0.2
Custard Tarts		277	6.3	32.4	14.5	1.2
Cyder Vinegar	Holland & Barrett	1.8	nil	0.4	nil	0.4

D

Product	*Brand*	*Calories kcal*	*Protein (g)*	*Carbo-hydrate (g)*	*Fat (g)*	*Dietary Fibre (g)*
Dairy Box Assortment	Nestlé Rowntree	478	5.7	60.8	23.5	0.8
Dairy/Fat Spread (see also brands & flavours)		662	0.4	Tr	73.4	nil
Dairy Fudge	Trebor Bassett	450	2.2	71.5	17.3	nil
Dairy Ice Cream: *see Ice Cream*						
Dairylea Cheese Food Slices	Kraft	305	13.0	8.0	24.5	nil
Light		220	18.5	7.0	12.5	nil
Dairylea Dip & Breadstick Dunkers, each	Kraft	157	4.9	13.5	9.3	0.5

All amounts given per 100g/100ml unless otherwise stated

Product	*Brand*	*Calories kcal*	*Protein (g)*	*Carbo-hydrate (g)*	*Fat (g)*	*Dietary Fibre (g)*
Dairylea Dip & Jumbo Chipsticks Dunkers, each	Kraft	4.1	13.5	12.5	13.5	0.7
Dairylea Dip & Pizza Crackers Dunkers, each	Kraft	188	5.3	12.5	13.5	0.7
Dairylea Double Cheese Lunchables, per pack	Kraft	415	19.5	19.0	29.0	0.4
Dairylea Harvest Ham Lunchables, per pack	Kraft	315	18.0	18.0	18.5	0.4
Dairylea Original Strip Cheese	Kraft	345	24.5	0.4	27.0	nil
Dairylea Pizza Flavour Strip Cheese	Kraft	350	23.5	1.0	26.5	0.1
Dairylea Portions	Kraft	270	9.1	8.6	22.0	nil
Dairylea Tasty Chicken Lunchables, per pack	Kraft	315	18.5	19.0	18.0	0.4

Dairylea Tender Turkey Lunchables, per pack	Kraft	305	17.6	20.0	17.0	0.6
Dairy Milk Chocolate	Cadbury	525	7.8	56.8	29.4	n/a
Dairy Milk Quick	Cadbury	530	7.7	56.6	30.4	n/a
Dairy Milk Tasters	Cadbury	520	7.7	57.0	29.2	n/a
Dairy Toffee	Cravens	472	1.8	75.3	18.3	nil
Damsons						
raw (weighed with stones)		34.0	0.5	8.6	Tr	1.6
stewed with sugar		107	1.3	26.9	0.1	1.5
Dandelion & Burdock	Idris	22.0	nil	5.4	Tr	n/a
	Top Deck	4.5	Tr	0.9	nil	n/a
Danish Blue Cheese		347	20.1	Tr	29.6	nil
Danish Brown Bread	Heinz Weight Watchers	213	10.4	39.2	1.7	9.6
Danish Malted Bread	Heinz Weight Watchers	238	10.9	45.3	1.4	6.9
Danish Pastries		374	5.8	51.3	17.6	1.6

All amounts given per 100g/100ml unless otherwise stated

Product	*Brand*	*Calories kcal*	*Protein (g)*	*Carbo-hydrate (g)*	*Fat (g)*	*Dietary Fibre (g)*
Danish Toaster Bread	Sunblest	232	8.9	45.4	1.6	2.1
Danish White Bread	Heinz Weight Watchers	233	9.2	46.2	1.3	2.8
	Sunblest	232	8.9	45.4	1.6	2.1
Dansak Classic Curry Sauce	Homepride	95.0	3.4	13.1	3.2	n/a
Dansak Curry Sauce	Uncle Ben's	108	1.9	10.8	6.2	n/a
Dark Brown Soft Sugar	Tate & Lyle	378	0.4	94.5	nil	nil
Dark Chocolate bar, organic	Green & Black's	571	10.0	51.0	37.0	nil
Dark Classico, each	Lyons Maid	135	1.5	13.5	8.5	n/a
Darkness	Cadbury	470	4.1	60.3	23.6	n/a
Dark Rye Ryvita, per slice	Ryvita	27.0	0.9	5.6	0.2	1.7
Dark Treacle Cookies	Heinz Weight Watchers	423	5.2	66.7	15.1	1.7
Dates, raw, weighed with stones		227	2.8	57.1	0.2	1.5
dried		268	2.3	68.1	0.4	3.4

chopped	Holland & Barrett	241	2.8	57.1	0.2	3.4
block	Whitworths	288	3.3	68.0	0.2	n/a
stoned	Whitworths	287	3.2	68.0	0.2	3.9
Deep Pan Pizza Bases	Napolina	298	8.5	56.0	4.4	n/a
Deep Pasta Bake, chicken & tomato	Findus	95.0	4.5	13.0	3.0	1.3
Delight Diet	Van den Bergh	228	3.6	1.6	23.0	nil
Delight Low Fat Spread	Van den Bergh	357	0.2	3.6	38.0	nil
Demerara Sugar		394	0.5	104.5	nil	nil
Derby Cheese		402	24.2	0.1	33.9	nil
Desiccated Coconut: ***see Coconut***						
Devon Custard	Ambrosia	103	2.7	16.4	3.0	0.1
low fat	Ambrosia	72.0	2.9	12.7	1.1	0.1
Dhansak Cooking Sauce	Sharwood	91.0	2.8	9.7	4.6	1.8
Diabetic Products (Boots, Dietade): ***see individual flavours***						

All amounts given per 100g/100ml unless otherwise stated

Product	*Brand*	*Calories kcal*	*Protein (g)*	*Carbo-hydrate (g)*	*Fat (g)*	*Dietary Fibre (g)*
Diced Pineapple	Holland & Barrett	276	2.5	67.9	1.3	8.1
Dietade (Applefords): ***see individual products***						
Diet Drinks: ***see individual flavours***						
Diet Ski Yogurt (Eden Vale): ***see individual flavours***						
Digestive Biscuit	Holland & Barrett	477	5.4	66.3	21.2	Tr
organic	Doves Farm	390	5.6	54.2	16.8	5.1
Digestive Biscuits						
chocolate		493	6.8	66.5	24.1	2.2
organic milk chocolate	Doves Farm	439	5.8	53.4	22.5	4.3
plain		471	6.3	68.6	20.9	2.2
organic plain	Doves Farm	428	5.8	51.4	22.1	6.4
Dinosaur Bites	McCain	189	3.5	27.5	7.2	n/a
Ditto	Tunnock's	457	4.3	62.8	22.8	n/a
Dolmio Pasta & Pasta Sauces: ***see individual flavours***						

Double Chocolate Cake Bites	Mr Kipling	422	6.7	42.9	22.8	n/a
Double Decker	Cadbury	465	5.2	64.9	20.7	n/a
Double Fudge Dream	Cadbury	495	6.3	61.4	25.2	n/a
Double Gloucester Cheese		405	24.6	0.1	34.0	nil
Doublemint Chewing Gum	Wrigley	306	nil	n/a	nil	nil
Doughnuts, jam		336	5.7	48.8	14.5	N
ring		397	6.1	47.2	21.7	N
Dream Topping						
standard	Bird's	690	6.7	32.5	58.5	0.5
sugar free		695	7.3	30.5	60.5	0.5
Dressed Crab	Young's	105	16.9	nil	14.2	nil
Dried Bananas	Holland & Barrett	221	3.1	53.7	0.8	9.5
Dried Fruit Salad	Holland & Barrett	185	3.1	40.9	1.0	8.0
	Whitworths	145	2.6	39.9	0.5	4.2
Dried Milk , skimmed, as sold		348	36.1	52.9	0.6	nil

All amounts given per 100g/100ml unless otherwise stated

Product	Brand	Calories kcal	Protein (g)	Carbo-hydrate (g)	Fat (g)	Dietary Fibre (g)
Drifter	Nestlé Rowntree	478	4.5	65.9	21.8	0.9
Drinking Chocolate, powder		366	5.5	77.4	6.0	N
made up with whole milk		90.0	3.4	10.6	4.1	Tr
made up with semi-skimmed milk		71.0	3.5	10.8	1.9	Tr
Dripping, beef		891	Tr	Tr	99.0	nil
Dry Ginger Ale	Schweppes	16.0	nil	3.8	nil	n/a
Duck						
meat only, roast		189	25.3	nil	9.7	nil
meat, fat & skin, roast		339	19.6	nil	29.0	nil
Dumplings		208	2.8	24.5	11.7	0.9
Dundee Cake	Lyons Cakes	309	3.8	58.1	6.6	n/a
Duo de Mousse Dessert	Chambourcy	185	4.3	18.3	10.6	0.4
Dutch Apple Tart	McVitie's	237	3.2	34.4	9.9	0.6
Dutch Cheese: ***see Edam, Gouda***						

E

Product	Brand	Calories kcal	Protein (g)	Carbo-hydrate (g)	Fat (g)	Dietary Fibre (g)
Easter Bakewells	Mr Kipling	429	3.9	62.6	17.9	n/a
Easter Egg Cakes	Lyons Cakes	454	5.4	54.3	23.5	n/a
Easy Cook White Rice, boiled		138	2.6	30.9	1.3	0.1
Eccles Cakes		475	3.9	59.3	26.4	1.6
Echo Margarine	Van den Bergh	720	Tr	0.1	80.0	nil
Eclairs, frozen		396	5.6	26.1	30.6	0.8
Economy Salad Cream	Burgess	283	1.2	7.5	27.3	nil

All amounts given per 100g/100ml unless otherwise stated

Product	Brand	Calories kcal	Protein (g)	Carbo-hydrate (g)	Fat (g)	Dietary Fibre (g)
Edam Cheese		333	26.0	Tr	25.4	nil
Egg Fried Rice		208	4.2	25.7	10.6	0.4
Egg Mayonnaise & Tomato Sandwiches, per pack	Boots Shapers	340	15.0	43.0	12.0	5.1
Eggplant: *see Aubergine*						
Eggs, chicken						
raw, whole		147	12.5	Tr	10.8	nil
raw, white only		36.0	9.0	Tr	Tr	nil
raw, yolk only		339	16.1	Tr	30.5	nil
boiled		147	12.5	Tr	10.8	nil
fried		179	13.6	Tr	13.9	nil
poached		147	12.5	Tr	10.8	nil
scrambled with milk		247	10.7	0.6	22.6	nil
Eggs, duck, raw, whole		163	14.3	Tr	11.8	nil
Egg Salad Sandwich with Salad Cream	Heinz Weight Watchers	155	6.9	21.0	4.8	0.9

Elmlea Double Cream	Van den Bergh	349	2.4	3.9	36.0	0.3
Elmlea Ready Whipped Cream	Van den Bergh	253	1.5	6.3	24.8	Tr
Elmlea Single Cream	Van den Bergh	148	3.1	4.6	13.0	0.2
Elmlea Whipping Cream	Van den Bergh	285	2.4	3.5	29.0	0.2
Energie	Jordans	384	9.5	70.3	10.5	7.4
English Apple Juice	Cawston Vale	42.0	0.1	10.8	Tr	n/a
English Cheddar Cheese		412	25.5	0.1	34.4	nil
English Broccoli & Stilton Soups of the World	Knorr	488	7.7	28.6	38.1	n/a
English Mustard	Colman's	187	7.0	19.0	9.3	1.6
Entenmann's Chocolate Fudge Cake	Hibernia Brands	361	4.4	51.8	15.1	09.
Evaporated Milk, whole		151	8.4	8.5	9.4	nil
full cream	Nestlé Ideal	160	8.2	11.5	9.0	nil
Everton Mints	Cravens	413	0.6	89.8	5.7	nil

All amounts given per 100g/100ml unless otherwise stated

Product	*Brand*	*Calories kcal*	*Protein (g)*	*Carbo-hydrate (g)*	*Fat (g)*	*Dietary Fibre (g)*
Exotic Fruit Torte	St Ivel	100	2.9	14.8	1.8	1.7
Extra Basil Pasta Sauce	Dolmio	58.0	0.8	7.8	2.7	n/a
Extra Chunky Vegetables Pasta Sauce	Dolmio	35.0	1.9	6.9	Tr	n/a
Extra Garlic Pasta Sauce	Dolmio	38.0	1.1	7.3	0.5	n/a
Extra Hot Curry Paste	Sharwood	332	4.3	12.6	29.4	5.3
Extra Peppermint Chewing Gum	Wrigley	165	nil	N	nil	nil
Extra Strong Spearmints	Trebor Bassett	396	0.4	98.7	Tr	nil
Extra Virgin Olive Oil	Napolina	828	nil	nil	92.0	nil
Extreme Duo	Nestlé	189	2.4	19.8	11.2	n/a

F

Product	*Brand*	*Calories kcal*	*Protein (g)*	*Carbo-hydrate (g)*	*Fat (g)*	*Dietary Fibre (g)*
Fab, each	Nestlé	83.0	0.5	13.7	2.8	n/a
Faggots		268	11.1	15.3	18.5	N
Family Steak & Kidney Deep Pie	Ross	270	7.2	23.9	16.7	1.0
Fancy Iced Cakes		407	3.8	68.8	14.9	N
Farmhouse Chicken & Leek Soup	Knorr	401	6.4	51.2	19.0	1.8

All amounts given per 100g/100ml unless otherwise stated

Product	*Brand*	*Calories kcal*	*Protein (g)*	*Carbo-hydrate (g)*	*Fat (g)*	*Dietary Fibre (g)*
Farmhouse Mince & Vegetables	Tyne Brand	74.0	5.9	6.7	2.6	n/a
Farmhouse Sausage Casserole Dry Cooking Mix	Colman's	313	11.0	63.0	1.3	n/a
Farmhouse Slices	Lyons Cakes	372	3.8	55.2	14.5	n/a
Farmhouse Vegetable Packet Soup	Batchelors	28	1.0	5.3	0.3	0.5
Farmhouse Wheatbran	Mornflake	213	14.1	26.8	5.5	36.4
Farmhouse White Bread	Hovis	228	9.0	44.6	1.5	2.3
Farmhouse Wholemeal Bread	Hovis	206	10.2	36.6	2.1	5.3
Farrows Marrowfat Peas	Batchelors	77.0	5.9	12.3	0.5	4.9
Fat Free French Vinaigrette Dressing	Kraft	47.0	0.1	10.5	Tr	0.2
Fennel, Florence, raw		12.0	0.9	1.8	0.2	2.4
boiled		11.0	0.9	1.5	0.2	2.3

Feta Cheese		250	15.6	1.5	20.2	nil
Fig Rolls	Jacob's	340	3.5	64.2	7.8	3.7
	Jacob's Vitalinea	339	3.7	68.2	5.8	3.8
Figs, dried		209	3.3	48.6	1.5	7.5
ready to eat		122	0.4	7.2	Tr	6.9
Figs in Syrup	Libby	88.0	n/a	n/a	Tr	n/a
Filet-O-Fish, each	McDonald's	389	16.5	40.7	17.7	1.1
Fillet of Haddock with Julienne Veg.	Ross	125	13.0	3.2	6.8	0.1
Fine Tasses	Nescafé	100	14.1	10.0	0.2	10.4
Finger Shortbread	McVitie's	525	6.1	63.1	27.1	2.0
Fish & Potato Bake	Ross	83.0	5.8	8.1	3.3	0.1
Fish & Tomato Gratin	Ross	120	7.3	9.3	6.2	0.4
Fish Cakes, fried		188	9.1	15.1	10.5	N
each	Birds Eye	172	11.4	15.2	7.3	0.9

All amounts given per 100g/100ml unless otherwise stated

Product	*Brand*	*Calories kcal*	*Protein (g)*	*Carbo-hydrate (g)*	*Fat (g)*	*Dietary Fibre (g)*
Fish fingers fried in oil		233	13.5	17.2	12.7	0.6
grilled		214	15.1	19.3	9.0	0.7
grilled	Birds Eye	178	12.1	16.4	7.1	0.5
	Ross	186	11.5	16.3	8.6	0.7
Fish in Pastry with Cheese	Birds Eye	213	9.4	17.0	11.9	0.9
Fish Mornay	Ross	137	6.6	11.8	7.3	0.5
Fish Paste		169	15.3	3.7	10.4	0.2
Fish Pie		102	8.0	12.3	3.0	0.7
Fish Portions in Crispy Crumb	Ross	206	10.9	19.2	9.8	0.8
Fish Shop Cod Fillets	Ross	76.0	17.4	nil	0.7	nil
Fish Shop Fish Fillets	Ross	257	11.8	20.1	14.6	0.6
Fish Shop Haddock Fillets	Ross	73.0	16.8	nil	0.6	nil
Fish Shop Plaice Fillets	Ross	120	10.3	21.0	0.4	0.9
Fish Steaks in Butter Sauce	Ross	93.0	9.4	2.9	4.9	0.1
Fish Steaks in Parsley Sauce	Ross	85.0	9.4	2.9	4.9	0.1

Fish Stock Cubes	Knorr	323	19.2	16.2	20.2	0.7
Five Alive Blackcurrant	Coca-Cola	62.0	Tr	15.3	nil	n/a
Citrus	Coca-Cola	50.0	Tr	12.0	nil	n/a
Orange Breakfast	Coca-Cola	46.0	nil	10.8	nil	n/a
Tropical	Coca-Cola	41.0	Tr	10.0	nil	nil
Very Berry	Coca-Cola	54.0	nil	13.2	nil	n/a
Five Fruit 'C'	Libby	40.0	0.1	10.0	Tr	Tr
Five Fruits Fruit Burst	Del Monte	53.0	0.2	12.4	Tr	n/a
Five Grain Crispbread	Primula	322	12.0	62.9	2.5	16.2
Flake	Cadbury	530	8.1	55.7	30.7	n/a
Flake Cakes	Cadbury	447	5.9	54.3	22.2	n/a
Flaky Pastry: ***see Pastry***						
Flapjacks		484	4.5	60.4	26.6	2.7
Flora Sunflower Oil	Van den Bergh	900	nil	nil	100	nil
Flora Sunflower Spread	Van den Bergh	630	0.1	0.1	70.0	nil
buttery	Van den Bergh	637	1.1	0.5	70.0	nil

All amounts given per 100g/100ml unless otherwise stated

Product	Brand	Calories kcal	Protein (g)	Carbo-hydrate (g)	Fat (g)	Dietary Fibre (g)
Flora Sunflower Spread (continued)						
light	Van den Bergh	357	0.1	3.7	38.0	0.6
low salt	Van den Bergh	630	0.1	0.1	70.0	nil
Florida Orange	Tunnock's	519	5.1	64.0	29.0	n/a
Florida Spring Vegetable Soup	Knorr	253	9.1	40.0	6.3	7.1
Flour, wheat						
brown		323	12.6	68.5	1.8	6.4
white, breadmaking		341	11.5	75.3	1.4	3.1
white, plain		341	9.4	77.7	1.3	3.1
white, self-raising		330	8.9	75.6	1.2	3.1
wholemeal		310	12.7	63.9	2.2	9.0
Forest Fruits Hot 'n' Fruity Custard Pot, each	Bird's	171	1.6	32.0	4.1	0.1
Four Cheese Dressing for Pasta	Crosse & Blackwell	240	3.1	8.8	21.1	0.3

Four Cheese Sauce	Colman's	400	18.0	38.0	18.0	n/a
Four Nut Country Crisp	Jordans	490	8.8	52.9	27.0	7.2
Fox's Glacier Fruits	Nestlé Rowntree	386	nil	96.7	nil	n/a
Fox's Glacier Mints	Nestlé Rowntree	386	nil	96.4	nil	n/a
Frankfurters		274	9.5	3.0	25.0	0.1
Freddo	Cadbury	525	7.8	56.8	29.4	
French Beans: ***see Green Beans/French Beans***						
French Bread Pizza: ***see individual flavours***						
French Dressing		649	0.3	0.1	72.1	nil
French Fancies	Mr Kipling	375	2.3	68.4	10.3	n/a
French Fries, regular, per portion	McDonald's	223	2.6	28.1	11.2	3.5
French Mix Vegetables	Ross	21.0	1.7	5.1	0.1	1.8
French Mustard	Burgess	145	7.5	14.9	4.9	0.6
	Colman's	104	6.3	4.0	7.0	3.8

All amounts given per 100g/100ml unless otherwise stated

Product	Brand	Calories kcal	Protein (g)	Carbo-hydrate (g)	Fat (g)	Dietary Fibre (g)
French Onion Soup	Baxters	22.0	0.7	4.2	0.2	0.4
	Knorr	315	8.2	62.0	3.8	7.4
French's Classic Yellow Mustard	Colman's	73.0	4.3	2.6	4.2	n/a
French Sandwich Cake	Lyons Cakes	356	3.9	54.0	12.7	n/a
Fresh Garden Mint Sauce	Colman's	30.0	1.4	2.6	0.1	n/a
Freshwater King Prawns	Lyons Seafoods	70.0	16.8	nil	0.3	n/a
Fried Bread: *see Bread, fried*						
Frijj Milkshakes, all varieties	Dairy Crest	64.0	3.3	12.7	0.8	n/a
Fromage frais						
fruit		131	6.8	13.8	5.8	Tr
plain		113	6.8	5.7	7.1	nil
very low fat		58.0	7.7	6.8	0.2	Tr
	Nestlé Smooth	165	6.4	16.5	8.3	0.1
Frosted Chex	Weetabix	375	6.1	83.7	1.7	3.5

Frosted Shreddies	Nestlé	363	7.2	80.5	1.4	6.1
Frosted Wheats	Kellogg's	340	10.0	72.0	1.5	9.0
Frosties	Kellogg's	370	5.0	88.0	0.5	2.0
Fruit 'n' Fibre	Kellogg's	350	9.0	69.0	4.5	9.0
Fruit & Nut Bran	Weetabix	319	12.6	49.3	8.0	18.3
Fruit & Nut Chocolate	Cadbury	490	8.0	55.7	26.3	n/a
Fruit &Nut Crunch	Holland & Barrett	372	10.1	61.1	11.2	6.7
Fruit & Nut Tasters	Cadbury	505	9.3	52.1	29.0	n/a
Fruit & Spice Pancakes	Sunblest	277	6.5	50.7	5.3	1.7
Fruit Burst Drinks (Del Monte): ***see individual flavours***						
Fruit Cake						
plain, retail		354	5.1	57.9	12.9	N
rich, recipe		341	3.8	59.6	11.0	1.7
rich, iced		356	4.1	62.7	11.4	1.7
wholemeal		363	6.0	52.8	15.7	2.4

All amounts given per 100g/100ml unless otherwise stated

Product	*Brand*	*Calories kcal*	*Protein (g)*	*Carbo-hydrate (g)*	*Fat (g)*	*Dietary Fibre (g)*
Fruit Club Biscuits	Jacob's	506	4.9	63.6	25.8	2.5
Fruit Cocktail						
canned in juice		57.0	0.4	14.8	Tr	1.0
	Del Monte	49.0	0.4	11.2	0.1	n/a
	Libby	52.0	0.2	12.7	Tr	0.3
canned in syrup		77.0	0.4	20.1	Tr	1.0
	Del Monte	75.0	0.4	18.0	0.1	n/a
	Libby	74.0	0.2	18.2	Tr	0.4
Fruit Cocktail Luxury Trifle	St Ivel	169	1.9	22.6	7.9	0.2
Fruit Cocktail Trifle	St Ivel	182	2.5	23.1	8.8	0.4
Fruit Drops	Cravens	386	2.0	70.3	22.7	0.5
Fruited Teacakes, each	Sunblest	211	5.0	37.3	4.6	1.5
Fruitetts	G. Payne & Co	395	Tr	92.7	27.0	n/a
Fruit Flapjack	Holland & Barrett	468	4.8	58.0	24.1	1.8

Fruit Gums		172	1.0	44.8	nil	nil
	Nestlé Rowntree	337	4.6	79.9	nil	nil
Fruitini Mixed Fruit Pieces in Custardy Banana Sauce	Del Monte	72.0	1.2	15.7	0.9	n/a
Fruitini Mixed Fruit Pieces in Orange Jelly	Del Monte	67.0	0.3	15.8	0.1	n/a
Fruitini Peaches in Juice	Del Monte	55.0	0.4	13.0	0.1	n/a
Fruitini Peach Pieces in Strawberry Jelly	Del Monte	65.0	0.3	15.3	0.1	n/a
Fruit Jaspers	McVitie's	499	5.4	65.6	23.6	3.4
Fruit Mousse		137	4.5	18.0	5.7	N
Fruit Pastil Lolly, each	Nestlé	57.0	nil	13.5	nil	n/a
Fruit Pastilles	Nestlé Rowntree	348	4.3	82.9	nil	nil
Fruit Pie, one crust		186	2.0	28.7	7.9	1.7
pastry top & bottom		260	3.0	34.0	13.3	1.8
individual		369	4.3	56.7	15.5	N
wholemeal, one crust		183	2.6	26.6	8.1	2.7

All amounts given per 100g/100ml unless otherwise stated

Product	*Brand*	*Calories kcal*	*Protein (g)*	*Carbo-hydrate (g)*	*Fat (g)*	*Dietary Fibre (g)*
Fruit Pies (Mr Kipling): ***see individual flavours***						
Fruit Salad Chews	Trebor Bassett	400	0.7	84.5	6.2	nil
Fruit Salad, homemade, dried		19.0	1.1	3.0	0.4	1.5
Fruit Shortcake	McVitie's	488	5.1	70.6	19.5	2.6
Fruit Trifles	Mr Kipling	392	3.4	52.3	17.8	n/a
Fruits o' Forest Bio Splitpot, per pack	Boots Shapers	79.0	n/a	n/a	0.2	n/a
Fruits of the Forest Cheesecake	McVitie's	302	4.5	31.9	17.7	0.6
Fruits of the Forest in Syrup	Libby	82.0	0.4	20.2	Tr	0.5
Fruits of the Forest Pavlova	McVitie's	293	2.7	43.6	12.0	Tr
Fruity Sauce	HP	141	1.2	35.1	0.1	n/a
Fry's Turkish Delight Cakes	Cadbury	371	4.5	62.4	10.8	n/a

Fudge	Cadbury	445	2.8	72.3	16.3	n/a
Funghi Pastaria Sauce	Knorr	520	6.9	45.7	34.4	1.4
Funghi Tastebreaks Pasta Snack	Knorr	436	10.1	61.0	17.0	n/a
Fuse	Cadbury	485	7.6	58.2	24.8	n/a

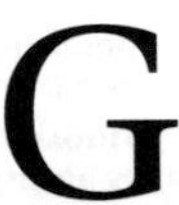

Product	*Brand*	*Calories kcal*	*Protein (g)*	*Carbo-hydrate (g)*	*Fat (g)*	*Dietary Fibre (g)*
Galaxy Caramel	Mars	488	5.3	60.1	25.1	n/a
Galaxy Caramel Egg	Mars	465	5.5	61.0	22.1	n/a
Galaxy Caramel Swirl Ice Cream	Mars	336	4.2	31.9	21.2	n/a
Galaxy Chocolate Swirls Ice Cream	Mars	331	4.1	33.2	20.3	n/a
Galaxy Double Nut/Raisin	Mars	534	8.4	55.7	30.8	n/a
Galaxy Hazelnut	Mars	572	7.7	48.5	38.6	n/a

All amounts given per 100g/100ml unless otherwise stated

Product	Brand	Calories kcal	Protein (g)	Carbo-hydrate (g)	Fat (g)	Dietary Fibre (g)
Galaxy Milk Chocolate Bar	Mars	488	5.3	60.1	25.1	n/a
Galaxy Minstrels	Mars	491	6.0	69.5	21.0	n/a
Galaxy Ripple	Mars	532	9.0	56.6	30.0	n/a
Galaxy Truffle Egg	Mars	586	5.1	52.0	39.7	n/a
Gammon: *see Bacon, gammon*						
Garden Peas	Birds Eye	62.0	4.9	9.0	0.7	4.5
	Ross	72.0	6.0	14.5	0.8	4.3
Garden Pea with Mint Soup	Baxters	32.0	1.6	6.3	0.3	1.8
Garlic, raw		98.0	7.9	16.3	0.6	4.1
Garlic & Black Pepper Cracker	Jacob's Vitalinea	399	11.7	74.2	6.1	4.6
Garlic & Butter Delicately Flavoured Rice	Batchelors	350	8.0	79.8	2.8	5.0
Garlic & Herb Chicken Marinade	Birds Eye	190	15.1	10.7	9.6	0.3

Garlic & Herb Cook-In-Sauce	Homepride	74.0	1.2	8.3	3.9	n/a
Garlic & Herb Dip, per pack	Primula	344	4.8	3.6	34.5	n/a
Garlic & Herb Light Reduced Calorie Salad Dressing	Hellmanns	237	0.6	13.9	19.4	n/a
Garlic &Herb Potato Bake	Homepride	234	1.0	1.7	24.8	n/a
Garlic & Herb Potato Roasters	Colman's	330	8.9	52.7	11.1	3.8
Garlic & Herb Sauce Mix, as sold	Colman's	413	13.0	47.0	19.0	n/a
Garlic & Italian Herbs for Pasta Seasoning Cubes	Knorr	278	10.3	5.2	24.0	1.1
Garlic Bites	Jacob's	529	7.5	53.7	31.6	2.0
Garlic Herb & Spice Cubes, each	Oxo	19.0	0.9	3.2	0.4	0.2
Garlic Mushroom Pasta Choice, as sold	Crosse & Blackwell	365	13.4	61.4	7.2	2.9
Garlic Prawnnaise	Lyons Seafoods	410	6.1	1.9	41.8	n/a

All amounts given per 100g/100ml unless otherwise stated

Product	Brand	Calories kcal	Protein (g)	Carbo-hydrate (g)	Fat (g)	Dietary Fibre (g)
Garlic Puree	Sharwood	63.0	3.4	13.3	0.3	2.4
Garlic Sauce	Lea & Perrins	337	1.8	17.8	29.0	n/a
Garlic Scooples	Kavli	341	11.5	76.8	1.9	7.4
Garlic Wholegrain Crispbread	Kavli	363	9.5	69.3	5.2	10.3
Gateau		337	5.7	43.4	16.8	0.4
Ghee						
butter		898	Tr	Tr	99.8	nil
palm		897	Tr	Tr	99.7	nil
vegetable		898	Tr	Tr	99.8	nil
Gherkins, pickled		14.0	0.9	2.6	0.1	1.2
raw		12.0	1.0	1.8	0.1	0.8
Giant Cornish Pastie	Ross	228	6.5	24.5	12.0	1.0
Giant Minced Beef & Onion Pastie	Ross	259	6.0	28.0	14.2	1.2
Giant Minestrone Soup	Heinz Big Soup	44.0	1.7	8.1	0.5	1.0

Gin: *see Spirits*						
Ginger & Zest Fruit Shorties	Jacob's Vitalinea	435	6.4	73.4	12.9	1.9
Ginger Beer	Idris	49.0	nil	12.1	nil	n/a
Gingernut Biscuits		456	5.6	79.1	15.2	1.4
	McVitie's	460	5.2	75.4	15.1	1.7
Ginger Root, raw		38.0	1.4	7.2	0.6	N
Ginger Sauce	Lea & Perrins	116	0.3	28.8	Tr	n/a
Gipsy Creams	McVitie's	514	4.9	62.8	26.9	2.6
Glacé Cherries: *see Cherries*						
Glacé Ginger	Whitworths	303	0.1	74.2	0.7	Tr
Glazed Chicken	Findus Lean Cuisine	90.0	6.0	12.5	1.5	0.8
Glazed Mince Tartlets	Mr Kipling	370	3.9	55.5	14.7	n/a
Glazed Chicken Platter, per meal	Birds Eye Healthy Options	345	32.0	32.0	9.5	4.0

All amounts given per 100g/100ml unless otherwise stated

Product	Brand	Calories kcal	Protein (g)	Carbo-hydrate (g)	Fat (g)	Dietary Fibre (g)
Globe Artichoke: ***see Artichoke, globe***						
Goats Milk		60.0	3.1	4.4	3.5	nil
Goats Milk Yogurt	Holland & Barrett	60.0	3.3	4.4	3.5	Tr
Gold Blend	Nescafé	95.0	13.3	10.0	0.2	18.0
decaffinated	Nescafé	110	14.5	12.0	0.2	11.6
Golden Calamari	Young's	299	13.7	15.8	20.4	0.7
Golden Churn	St Ivel	642	0.9	2.4	70.0	nil
Golden Garlic Prawns	Young's	223	10.0	19.6	12.0	0.8
Golden Grahams	Nestlé	381	5.6	81.6	3.6	3.2
Golden Hake Fillets	Ross	256	9.0	17.4	17.0	0.7
Golden King Prawns	Young's	241	8.7	15.6	16.3	0.7
Golden Lemon Sole Goujons	Young's	246	10.9	26.4	11.2	1.1
Golden Prawn Nuggets	Young's	175	11.5	11.1	9.6	0.5

Golden Savoury Rice	Batchelors	364	10.1	74.7	2.8	2.4
Golden Scampi in Breadcrumbs	Young's	172	9.4	22.1	5.5	0.9
Golden Syrup		298	0.3	79.0	nil	nil
	Lyle's	325	0.5	80.5	nil	nil
Golden Syrup Oatso Simple	Quaker	364	7.5	70.0	5.5	5.0
Golden Vegetable Cup-A-Soup, per sachet	Batchelors	70.0	1.0	15.3	0.5	0.9
Golden Vegetable Rice	Birds Eye	112	3.5	23.7	0.4	1.4
Golden Vegetable Slim-A-Soup, per sachet	Batchelors	58.0	1.1	9.7	1.7	1.5
Golden Vegetable Soup	Knorr	345	10.3	57.8	8.0	3.3
per pack	Boots Shapers	40.00	n/a	n/a	1.1	n/a
Golden Whitebait	Young's	338	13.3	17.1	24.4	0.7
Gold Light Margarine	St Ivel	365	2.8	2.9	38.0	Tr
lowest fat	St Ivel	259	0.6	3.4	27.0	Tr
unsalted	St Ivel	360	0.7	3.9	38.0	Tr

All amounts given per 100g/100ml unless otherwise stated

Product	Brand	Calories kcal	Protein (g)	Carbo-hydrate (g)	Fat (g)	Dietary Fibre (g)
Goose, roast, meat only		319	29.3	nil	22.4	nil
Gooseberries						
raw		54.0	0.7	12.9	0.3	2.4
stewed with sugar		73.0	0.4	18.5	0.2	2.0
green, stewed without sugar		16.0	0.9	2.5	0.3	1.9
Gooseberry Custard Style Yogurt	Boots Shapers	51.0	n/a	n/a	0.8	n/a
Gouda Cheese		375	24.0	Tr	31.0	nil
Gourmet King Prawns	Lyons Seafoods	51.0	12.0	nil	0.5	n/a
Granary Bread: *see Bread*						
Granary Brown Bread	Hovis	225	9.1	42.7	2.0	3.3
Grannies Cake	Lyons Cakes	410	4.4	50.2	21.2	n/a
Granulated Sugar	Tate & Lyle	400	nil	99.9	nil	nil
Grapefruit, raw, flesh only		30.0	0.8	6.8	0.1	1.3
canned in juice		30.0	0.6	7.3	Tr	0.4

canned in syrup		60.0	0.5	15.5	Tr	0.6
Grapefruit & Orange in Syrup	Libby	77.0	0.5	18.8	Tr	0.3
Grapefruit 'C'	Libby	36.0	0.2	8.8	Tr	0.3
Grapefruit Juice, unsweetened		33.0	0.4	8.3	0.1	Tr
	Britvic	40.0	0.5	8.1	0.1	n/a
	Del Monte	41.0	0.5	8.8	Tr	n/a
Grapefruit Segments in Syrup	Libby	78.0	0.5	18.9	Tr	0.3
Grapefruit with Apple Juice	Cawston Vale	42.0	0.2	10.6	Tr	n/a
Grape Juice, unsweetened		46.0	0.3	11.7	0.1	nil
red, sparkling	Schloer	49.0	Tr	13.1	n/a	n/a
white	Schloer	48.0	Tr	12.9	n/a	n/a
white, sparkling	Schloer	49.0	Tr	13.1	n/a	n/a
Grape Nuts	Bird's	345	10.5	72.5	1.9	8.6
Grapes, black/white, seedless		60.0	0.4	15.4	0.1	0.7

All amounts given per 100g/100ml unless otherwise stated

Product	*Brand*	*Calories kcal*	*Protein (g)*	*Carbo-hydrate (g)*	*Fat (g)*	*Dietary Fibre (g)*
Gravy Browning	Burgess	72.0	3.3	14.7	nil	nil
	Crosse & Blackwell	192	Tr	48.0	nil	nil
Gravy Instant Granules		462	4.4	40.6	32.5	Tr
made up with water		33.0	0.3	2.9	2.4	Tr
Greek Pastries (sweet)		322	4.7	40.0	17.0	N
Greek Style Raspberry Yogurt, per pack	Boots Shapers	126	n/a	n/a	4.5	n/a
Greek Style Strawberry Yogurt, per pack	Boots Shapers	130	n/a	n/a	4.5	n/a
Greek Style Vanilla Yogurt, per pack	Boots Shapers	126	n/a	n/a	4.5	n/a
Greek Yogurt: *see Yogurt*						
Green Beans/French Beans						
raw		24.0	1.9	3.2	0.5	2.2
boiled		22.0	1.8	2.9	0.5	2.4

frozen, boiled		25.0	1.7	4.7	0.1	4.1
canned		22.0	1.5	4.1	0.1	2.6
Green Butterfly	Fussell's	160	8.2	11.5	9.0	nil
Green Chilli & Garlic Poppadums	Sharwood	274	19.9	43.3	1.6	9.7
Greengages						
raw (weighed with stones)		34.0	0.5	8.6	Tr	1.6
stewed with sugar		107	1.3	26.9	0.1	1.5
Green Label Chutney Sauce	Sharwood	222	1.0	44.8	0.3	1.4
Green Lentils: *see Lentils*						
Green Peppers: *see Peppers*						
Greens, spring: *see Spring Greens*						
Grillsteaks, grilled		305	22.1	0.5	23.9	Tr
	Ross	315	15.9	nil	28.0	ni
Groundnuts: *see Peanuts*						
Ground Rice	Whitworths	361	6.5	86.8	1.0	0.5

All amounts given per 100g/100ml unless otherwise stated

Product	*Brand*	*Calories kcal*	*Protein (g)*	*Carbo-hydrate (g)*	*Fat (g)*	*Dietary Fibre (g)*
Grouse, roast		173	31.3	nil	5.3	nil
Guavas						
raw		26.0	0.8	5.0	0.5	3.7
canned in syrup		60.0	0.4	15.7	Tr	n/a
Gumbo: ***see Okra***						

H

Product	*Brand*	*Calories kcal*	*Protein (g)*	*Carbo-hydrate (g)*	*Fat (g)*	*Dietary Fibre (g)*
Haddock						
steamed, flesh only		98.0	22.8	nil	0.8	nil
in crumbs, fried in oil		174	21.4	3.6	8.3	0.2
smoked, steamed, flesh only		101	23.3	nil	0.9	nil
Haddock & Prawn Crumble	Ross	181	8.7	12.6	11.2	0.5
Haddock Bake	Ross	142	7.7	11.9	7.3	0.5
Haddock Fillet Fish Fingers	Birds Eye	167	12.4	13.2	7.2	0.9
Haddock Steaks in Butter Sauce	Ross	90.0	10.2	2.9	4.2	0.1

All amounts given per 100g/100ml unless otherwise stated

Product	*Brand*	*Calories kcal*	*Protein (g)*	*Carbo-hydrate (g)*	*Fat (g)*	*Dietary Fibre (g)*
Haddock Steaks in Crispy Crunch Crumb, each	Birds Eye	225	14.0	13.0	13.0	0.9
Haddock Steaks in Natural Crumb	Ross	189	11.2	13.4	10.3	0.6
Haggis, boiled		310	10.7	19.2	21.7	N
Halibut, steamed, flesh only		131	23.8	nil	4.0	nil
Ham, canned		120	18.4	nil	5.1	nil
Ham & Beef Spread	Shippams	180	15.7	2.9	11.7	n/a
Ham & Cheese Soup	Campbell's	59.0	1.3	3.3	4.5	n/a
Ham & Cheese Toast Topper	Heinz	96.0	7.4	7.3	4.1	0.1
Ham & Edam with Salad and Mayonnaise Sandwich, per pack	Boots Shapers	303	18.0	33.0	11.0	5.3
Ham & Leek Potato Bake	Colman's	412	9.9	40.4	24.0	2.1
Ham & Mushroom French Bread Pizza	Findus	180	7.3	26.5	5.1	2.0

Ham & Mushroom Pizza	San Marco	227	11.4	29.5	7.5	1.1
5"	McCain	184	8.7	27.7	4.3	n/a
Ham & Pineapple French Bread Pizza	Findus	190	7.3	28.5	5.0	1.4
Ham & Pineapple 95% Fat Free Dip	St Ivel Shape	88.0	7.0	5.9	4.0	Tr
Ham & Pork, chopped, canned		275	14.4	1.4	23.6	0.3
Hamburger, each	McDonald's	253	13.1	32.8	7.7	2.5
Hamburger Buns		264	9.1	48.8	5.0	1.5
Ham Sandwich Filler	Heinz	198	5.4	11.0	14.7	0.5
Ham, Soft Cheese & Pineapple Sandwiches, per pack	Boots Shapers	295	18.0	34.0	9.7	4.7
Ham Stock Cubes	Knorr	309	11.2	23.5	18.9	nil
Hard Cheese, average		405	24.7	0.1	34.0	nil
Haricot Beans, dried, boiled		95.0	6.6	17.2	0.5	6.1
Harvest Luxury Raisin Crunch	Quaker	430	6.5	65.5	15.5	5.0

All amounts given per 100g/100ml unless otherwise stated

Product	*Brand*	*Calories kcal*	*Protein (g)*	*Carbo-hydrate (g)*	*Fat (g)*	*Dietary Fibre (g)*
Harvest Nut Crunch	Quaker	459	8.0	62.5	19.5	6.0
Harvest Tropical Crunch	Quaker	437	6.5	64.0	17.0	6.0
Hash Browns	McCain	190	3.0	24.0	9.8	n/a
	McDonald's	127	1.2	14.1	7.3	2.1
Hawaiian Crunch	Mornflake	414	8.0	68.3	12.1	5.6
Hazelnut & Currant Chocolate, organic	Green & Black's	528	7.7	49.7	34.5	nil
Hazlenut Chocolate Multipack, per pack	Boots Shapers	218	n/a	n/a	5.1	n/a
Hazelnut Dessert (in pots)	Provamel	101	3.0	16.0	2.8	1.2
Hazelnuts, kernel only		650	14.1	6.0	63.5	6.5
Healthy Baked Beans	HP	63.0	4.4	11.0	0.2	3.7
Healthy Balance Baked Beans & Vegetable Sausages	Heinz	96.0	5.8	10.2	3.6	2.9

Healthy Balance Baked Beans in Tomato Sauce	Heinz	67.0	4.6	11.7	0.2	3.7
Heart						
ox, stewed		179	31.4	nil	5.9	nil
sheep, roast		237	26.1	nil	14.7	nil
Hearty Minestrone	Campbell's	21.0	0.5	4.5	0.1	n/a
Hearty Vegetable	Campbell's	27.0	0.8	5.5	0.3	n/a
Herb & Garlic Pâté	Tartex	230	7.5	10.0	18.0	n/a
Herb & Tomato Mustard	Colman's	228	9.5	26.0	8.5	3.6
Herb Pâté	Tartex	230	7.0	10.0	18.5	n/a
per tub	Vessen	109	3.1	5.4	8.0	0.1
Heroes	Cadbury	505	6.0	61.3	26.3	n/a
Herring						
raw		234	16.8	nil	18.5	nil
fried, flesh only		234	23.1	1.5	15.1	N
grilled, flesh only		199	20.4	nil	13.0	nil

All amounts given per 100g/100ml unless otherwise stated

Product	*Brand*	*Calories kcal*	*Protein (g)*	*Carbo-hydrate (g)*	*Fat (g)*	*Dietary Fibre (g)*
HiBran Bread	Allinson	219	12.6	35.0	3.2	6.8
Hickory Nuts: *see Pecan Nuts*						
Hi-Fibre Biscuits	Itona	316	9.4	43.2	11.7	10.0
Hi-Fibre Biscuits with Date Syrup	Itona	387	10.3	48.2	18.5	12.3
High Bake Water Biscuits	Jacob's	412	9.8	76.3	7.5	3.2
High Fibre Muesli	Holland & Barrett	317	10.3	70.9	1.8	5.9
High Juice Orange, per pack	Boots Shapers	42.0	n/a	n/a	Tr	n/a
Highlander's Broth	Baxters	43.0	1.6	6.1	1.4	0.5
Hi-Juice 66	Schweppes	52.0	2.17	12.2	nil	n/a
Hilo Crackers	Rakusen	349	11.0	74.0	1.0	8.0
Hippo Fromage Frais Dessert, all flavours	Chambourcy	125	6.8	14.8	4.5	0.1

Hob Nob Bars	McVitie's	523	6.4	61.6	27.9	2.8
Hoi Sin Chinese Spare Rib Sauce	Sharwood	182	2.8	38.3	2.4	1.9
Hollandaise Sauce Dry Mix, as sold	Crosse & Blackwell	390	10.0	50.3	16.8	1.6
Honey, comb		281	0.6	74.4	4.6	nil
in jars		288	0.4	76.4	nil	nil
	Holland & Barrett	307	0.4	76.5	0.1	nil
Honey & Almond Crunchy Bar, each	Jordans	155	2.9	18.7	7.6	1.9
Honey & Mustard Chicken Tonight Sauce	Batchelors	107	1.6	13.5	5.2	1.3
Honey Bran Oatso Simple	Quaker	352	8.5	65.0	6.0	6.0
Honeycomb: *see Honey, comb*						
Honeydew Melon: *see Melon*						
Honey Nut Cheerios	Nestlé	383	8.6	77.0	4.6	3.5

All amounts given per 100g/100ml unless otherwise stated

Product	*Brand*	*Calories kcal*	*Protein (g)*	*Carbo-hydrate (g)*	*Fat (g)*	*Dietary Fibre (g)*
Honey Nut Loops	Kellogg's	370	8.0	77.0	3.0	7.0
Honey Rice Krispies	Kellogg's	380	4.5	89.0	0.7	1.0
Honey Rich Baste 'n' Grill Sauce	Lea & Perrins	177	2.1	40.6	0.9	n/a
Hong Kong Black Pepper Sauce	Amoy	142	2.2	20.5	5.7	n/a
Horlicks Light Chocolate Malt Drink	SmithKline Beecham	390	9.0	71.6	7.5	5.6
Horlicks Light Hot Chocolate Drink	SmithKline Beecham	399	8.8	72.6	8.1	3.7
Horlicks Light Instant Powder	SmithKline Beecham	381	13.7	71.5	4.5	2.7
made up with water		122	4.4	22.3	1.4	0.9
Horlicks Powder		381	9.6	75.0	4.7	4.0
made up with whole milk		222	7.4	27.9	9.2	1.0

made up with semi-skimmed milk		181	7.7	28.3	4.5	1.0
Horseradish Mustard	Colman's	185	6.5	22.0	7.2	3.3
Horseradish Sauce		153	2.5	17.9	8.4	2.5
	Baxters	326	2.9	5.6	32.5	nil
	Colman's	105	1.8	9.7	5.7	n/a
Hot & Spicy Chinese Chicken, per meal	Birds Eye	505	18.0	89.0	8.4	2.3
Hot 'n' Spicy Prawns	Lyons Seafoods	275	6.5	32.1	14.3	n/a
Hot Chicken Curry	Shippams	120	10.4	7.1	5.6	n/a
Hot Chicken Curry Pot Noodle	Golden Wonder	433	11.4	62.6	15.2	3.3
Hot Chilli Chinese Pouring Sauce	Sharwood	120	0.5	29.4	0.6	1.3
Hot Cross Buns		310	7.4	58.5	6.8	1.7
Hot Curry Paste	Sharwood	346	5.5	12.6	30.4	6.8
Hot Dog Spread	Primula	222	13.5	6.0	16.0	n/a

All amounts given per 100g/100ml unless otherwise stated

Product	*Brand*	*Calories kcal*	*Protein (g)*	*Carbo-hydrate (g)*	*Fat (g)*	*Dietary Fibre (g)*
Hot Horseradish Sauce	Burgess	131	2.2	14.1	6.7	2.0
Hot Pepperoni French Bread Pizza	Findus	200	7.2	26.7	7.2	1.5
Hot Pot		114	9.4	10.1	4.5	1.2
Hot Salsa	Heinz	30.0	1.7	5.5	0.2	1.4
Hot Salsa Dip	Primula	35.0	1.8	6.6	0.2	n/a
Houmous: *see Hummus*						
Hovis Bread: *see types of bread*						
Hovis Cracker	Jacob's	454	10.0	62.0	19.0	3.0
Hovis Digestive	Jacob's	473	7.7	67.0	19.3	2.3
HP Sauce	HP	119	0.9	27.5	0.2	n/a
Hubba Bubba Bubble Gum, all flavours	Wrigley	280	nil	n/a	nil	nil

Hula Hoops: ***see Potato Hoops***					
Hummus	187	7.6	11.6	12.6	2.4

All amounts given per 100g/100ml unless otherwise stated

I

Product	*Brand*	*Calories kcal*	*Protein (g)*	*Carbo-hydrate (g)*	*Fat (g)*	*Dietary Fibre (g)*
I Can't Believe It's Not Butter	Van den Bergh	625	0.4	0.7	69.0	nil
light	Van den Bergh	357	0.2	3.6	38.0	0.6
Ice by Tizer	Barr	40.0	Tr	9.6	Tr	nil
Ice Cream						
dairy, vanilla		194	3.6	24.4	9.8	Tr
dairy, flavoured		179	3.5	24.7	8.0	Tr
non-dairy, vanilla		178	3.2	23.1	8.7	Tr
non-dairy, flavoured		166	3.1	23.2	7.4	Tr
mixes		182	4.1	25.1	7.9	Tr

All amounts given per 100g/100ml unless otherwise stated

Product	Brand	Calories kcal	Protein (g)	Carbo-hydrate (g)	Fat (g)	Dietary Fibre (g)
Ice Cream Wafers		342	10.1	78.8	0.7	N
Iced Gem	Jacob's	403	5.4	88.5	5.4	1.5
Iced Strawberry Delights	Mr Kipling	378	3.4	58.6	14.0	n/a
Icing Sugar	Tate & Lyle	398	nil	99.5	nil	nil
Inchs White Lightning	H P Bulmer	52	n/a	n/a	n/a	n/a
Indian Chevda	Sharwood	523	7.1	44.3	36.5	7.2
Indian Chicken Balti Mix, as sold	Crosse & Blackwell	340	10.6	57.7	7.5	5.6
Indian Chicken Korma Mix, as sold	Crosse & Blackwell	345	10.2	49.8	11.2	5.0
Indian Chicken Stir Fry Meal	Ross	74.0	5.8	15.2	0.6	3.7
Indian Curry & Vegetables Stir Fry Sauce	Uncle Ben's	74.0	1.0	13.3	1.9	n/a
Indian Korma Make a Meal	Birds Eye	64.0	4.2	8.2	1.6	1.0

Indian Herb & Spice Cubes, each	Oxo	19.0	0.7	2.9	0.5	0.4
Indian Rices of the World	Batchelors	358	8.9	75.6	2.2	2.6
Indian Special Rice	Ross	118	2.8	26.1	0.8	1.3
Indian Tandoori Prawns Stir Fry	Ross	67.0	3.8	11.6	1.6	2.1
Indian Tikka Masala Cooking Sauce	Heinz Weight Watchers	55.0	1.4	8.6	1.7	0.8
Inspirations	Cadbury	500	6.1	55.6	28.0	n/a
Instant Coffee: ***see Coffee***						
Instant Creamy Mashed Potatoes, made up	Yeoman	60.0	1.6	12.9	0.2	n/a
Instant Dessert Powder		391	2.4	60.1	17.3	1.0
made up with whole milk		111	3.1	14.8	6.3	0.2
made up with skimmed milk		84.0	3.1	14.9	3.2	0.2
Instant Milk: ***see brands***						
Instant Potato Powder made up with water		57.0	1.5	13.5	0.1	1.0

All amounts given per 100g/100ml unless otherwise stated

Product	Brand	Calories kcal	Protein (g)	Carbo-hydrate (g)	Fat (g)	Dietary Fibre (g)
Instant Potato Powder (continued)						
made up with whole milk		76.0	2.4	14.8	1.2	1.0
made up with semi-skimmed milk		70.0	2.4	14.8	1.2	1.0
made up with skimmed milk		66.0	2.4	14.8	0.1	1.0
Instant Soup Powder, dried		341	6.5	64.4	14.0	N
made up with water		55.0	1.1	10.5	2.3	N
Irish Stew		123	5.3	9.1	7.6	0.9
	Tyne Brand	89.0	4.3	9.4	3.8	n/a
Irn Bru	Barr	41.0	Tr	10.1	Tr	nil
diet	Barr	0.7	Tr	Tr	Tr	nil
Italian & Garlic Vinaigrette Dressing	Kraft	128	0.4	7.2	10.5	0.2
Italian Bean & Pasta Soup	Baxters	38.0	1.9	7.0	0.2	1.3
Italian Bites	Jacob's	474	8.3	55.2	24.4	4.2
Italian Chicken Pasta Pot Light	Golden Wonder	327	15.3	62.0	1.9	5.3

Italian Herbs & Garlic Pasta 'n' Sauce	Batchelors	351	13.1	69.0	2.5	3.8
Italian Minestrone Soup of the World	Knorr	343	12.3	64.2	4.1	n/a
Italiano Fish Bake	Birds Eye	88.0	11.5	3.6	3.1	0.3
Italian Herb & Stock Cubes, each	Oxo	20.0	0.8	3.2	0.5	0.3
Italian Pasta Cooking Sauce	Heinz Weight Watchers	38.0	1.5	7.6	0.2	0.9
Italian Supernoodles	Batchelors	479	10.0	63.7	20.7	3.3
Italian Tomato &Basil Soup	Campbell's	68.0	1.0	5.3	4.8	n/a
Italian Tomato & Basil Tastebreaks Soup	Knorr	435	10.9	60.6	16.6	n/a
Italian Tomato & Mozzarella Chicken Lattice, each	Birds Eye	425	18.0	34.0	24.0	3.0
Italian Tomato with Penne Pasta Soup	Baxters	36.0	1.2	7.3	0.2	1.0

All amounts given per 100g/100ml unless otherwise stated

J

Product	*Brand*	*Calories kcal*	*Protein (g)*	*Carbo-hydrate (g)*	*Fat (g)*	*Dietary Fibre (g)*
Jacket Potato Cheese & Onion, half	Birds Eye	150	5.2	23.0	4.4	2.1
Jacket Scallopes	Ross	127	2.9	21.2	3.4	1.8
Jackfruit, raw		88.0	1.3	21.4	0.3	N
canned, drained		104	0.5	26.3	0.3	N
Jaffa Cakes	McVitie's	376	3.9	72.3	8.2	0.9
Jaffa Fingers	Lyons Cakes	476	3.6	62.7	23.4	n/a
Jaggery		367	0.5	97.2	nil	nil

All amounts given per 100g/100ml unless otherwise stated

Product	*Brand*	*Calories kcal*	*Protein (g)*	*Carbo-hydrate (g)*	*Fat (g)*	*Dietary Fibre (g)*
Jalfrezi Sizzle & Stir Sauce	Batchelors	109	1.1	5.0	9.4	2.4
Jam & Creamed	Jacob's Vitalinea	359	5.3	52.9	14.0	1.3
Jam						
fruit with edible seeds		261	0.6	69.0	nil	N
stone fruit		261	0.4	69.3	nil	N
reduced sugar		123	0.5	31.9	0.1	N
Jam Doughnuts: ***see Doughnuts***						
Jam Roly Poly	McVitie's	391	5.1	51.6	18.7	1.2
Jam Tarts, recipe		380	3.3	62.0	14.9	1.6
retail		368	3.3	63.4	13.0	N
assorted	Mr Kipling	401	3.5	64.1	14.5	n/a
Jamaica Ginger Bar Cake	McVitie's	380	4.1	55.8	14.8	0.9
Japanese Beef Oriental Stir Fry	Ross	62.0	5.4	9.4	1.0	1.5

Japanese Rice Crackers	Holland & Barrett	397	9.0	79.7	4.7	0.3
Jelly, made with water		61.0	1.2	15.1	nil	nil
Jelly Crystals: *see individual flavours*						
Jellytots	Nestlé Rowntree	346	0.1	86.5	nil	nil
Juicy Fruit Chewing Gum	Wrigley	295	nil	N	nil	nil
Jumbo Oats	Mornflake	364	11.8	62.0	7.6	7.2
Just Fruit Pastilles	Trebor Bassett	344	4.0	81.2	Tr	Tr
Just Right	Kellogg's	360	8.0	76.0	3.0	5.0

All amounts given per 100g/100ml unless otherwise stated

K

Product	Brand	Calories kcal	Protein (g)	Carbo-hydrate (g)	Fat (g)	Dietary Fibre (g)
Kale: ***see Curly Kale***						
Kashmir Mild Curry Sauce Mix	Sharwood	242	10.3	29.0	9.4	16.4
Kedgeree		166	14.2	10.5	7.9	Tr
Keg Bitter: ***see Beer***						
Ketchup, tomato		98.0	2.1	24.0	Tr	0.9
Kidney						
lamb, fried		155	24.6	nil	6.3	nil
ox, stewed		172	25.6	nil	7.7	nil

All amounts given per 100g/100ml unless otherwise stated

Product	*Brand*	*Calories kcal*	*Protein (g)*	*Carbo-hydrate (g)*	*Fat (g)*	*Dietary Fibre (g)*
Kidney (continued)						
pig, stewed		153	24.4	nil	6.1	nil
Kidney Beans: ***see Red Kidney Beans***						
King Banana, each	Lyons Maid	140	0.8	12.0	9.9	n/a
King Cones (Lyons Maid): ***see individual flavours***						
Kingsmill Country Gold Malted WheatBread	Allied Bakeries	234	9.4	43.4	2.5	2.7
Kingsmill White Bread	Allied Bakeries	233	8.8	44.1	2.4	2.5
Kingsmill White Rolls, each	Allied Bakeries	145	6.4	27.4	1.1	1.3
Kingsmill Wholemeal Gold	Allied Bakeries	221	10.9	37.8	2.9	6.0
Kipper Fillets with Butter	Birds Eye	205	15.0	nil	16.0	nil
Kippers, baked, flesh only		205	25.5	nil	11.4	nil
Kit Kat	Nestlé Rowntree	507	6.8	60.2	26.5	1.2
Kit Kat Chunky	Nestlé Rowntree	514	6.5	59.8	27.6	1.0

Kiwi & Lime Spring Water	Boots Shapers	1.0	n/a	n/a	Tr	n/a
Kiwi Fruit		49.0	1.1	10.6	0.5	1.9
Kiwi Fruit in Syrup	Libby	69.0	n/a	n/a	Tr	n/a
Kohlrabi, raw		23.0	1.6	3.7	0.2	2.2
boiled		18.0	1.2	3.1	0.2	1.9
Kola Chew Bar	Trebor Bassett	398	0.7	84.3	6.0	Tr
Kola Cubes	Cravens	386	Tr	96.4	nil	nil
each	Trebor Bassett	385	Tr	95.2	nil	nil
Korma Classic Curry Sauce	Homepride	69.0	1.3	11.6	2.0	n/a
Korma Curry Sauce	Sharwood	88.0	2.2	8.5	5.0	2.3
Korma Low in Fat Sauce	Homepride	57.0	1.2	9.1	1.8	n/a
Korma Sizzle & Stir Sauce	Batchelors	233	2.0	9.8	20.6	3.0
Krackawheat	McVitie's	518	8.3	61.0	25.8	4.9
Krispen Crispbread Crackers						
Light	Kavli	371	10.7	71.8	4.6	5.0
Rye	Kavli	272	10.5	53.0	2.0	21.0
Wholemeal Light	Kavli	366	9.7	71.2	4.7	7.9

All amounts given per 100g/100ml unless otherwise stated

Product	*Brand*	*Calories kcal*	*Protein (g)*	*Carbo-hydrate (g)*	*Fat (g)*	*Dietary Fibre (g)*
Krona Gold	Van den Bergh	632	0.2	0.3	70.0	nil
Krona 63% Fat Spread	Van den Bergh	569	0.2	0.3	63.0	nil

L

Product	Brand	Calories kcal	Protein (g)	Carbo-hydrate (g)	Fat (g)	Dietary Fibre (g)
Lady's Fingers: ***see Okra***						
Lager, bottled		29.0	0.2	1.5	Tr	nil
Lamb, breast						
lean & fat, roast		410	19.1	nil	37.1	nil
lean only, roast		252	25.6	nil	16.6	nil
Lamb, chops						
loin, lean & fat, grilled		355	23.5	nil	29.0	nil
loin, lean only, grilled		222	27.8	nil	12.3	nil

All amounts given per 100g/100ml unless otherwise stated

Product	Brand	Calories kcal	Protein (g)	Carbo-hydrate (g)	Fat (g)	Dietary Fibre (g)
Lamb, cutlets						
lean & fat, grilled		370	23.0	nil	30.9	nil
lean only, grilled		222	27.8	nil	12.3	nil
Lamb, leg						
lean & fat, roast		266	26.1	nil	17.9	nil
lean only, roast		191	29.4	nil	8.1	nil
Lamb, scrag & neck						
lean & fat, stewed		292	25.6	nil	21.1	nil
lean only, stewed		253	27.8	nil	15.7	nil
Lamb, shoulder						
lean & fat, roast		316	19.9	nil	26.3	nil
lean only, roast		196	23.8	nil	11.2	nil
Lamb Curry	Tyne Brand	99.0	6.1	7.2	5.1	n/a
with rice, per pack	Birds Eye	520	21.0	80.0	13.0	3.4
Lamb Grillsteak, each	Birds Eye	170	14.0	1.6	12.0	0.6
Lamb Hotpot	Heinz Baked Bean Cuisine	99.0	5.4	12.1	3.2	2.1

Lamb Hotpot Casserole Mix, as sold	Colman's	277	5.9	58.0	2.1	n/a
Lamb Moussaka	Heinz Weight Watchers	79.0	3.6	10.9	2.3	0.8
Lamb Oxo Cubes	Oxo	289	16.2	42.8	5.9	2.1
Lamb Ragout Classic Creations Mix, as sold	Crosse & Blackwell	340	9.5	59.9	6.9	1.9
Lamb Stock Cubes	Knorr	295	12.4	16.1	20.1	0.2
Lancashire Cheese		373	23.3	0.1	31.0	nil
Lancashire Hotpot	Tyne Brand	77.0	4.5	7.2	3.3	n/a
Lard		891	Tr	Tr	99.0	nil
Large Prunes	Holland & Barrett	134	2.0	33.5	Tr	13.4
Lasagne, frozen, cooked		102	5.0	12.8	3.8	N
	Chef	90.0	3.9	11.1	3.4	0.6
	Birds Eye	112	6.1	11.6	4.6	0.7
	Findus Pasta Choice	120	6.3	10.7	5.7	0.7

All amounts given per 100g/100ml unless otherwise stated

Product	*Brand*	*Calories kcal*	*Protein (g)*	*Carbo-hydrate (g)*	*Fat (g)*	*Dietary Fibre (g)*
Lasagne, frozen, cooked	Findus Red Box	115	6.4	10.4	5.3	0.7
Lasagne (pasta), dry						
egg	Buitoni	356	14.0	66.0	4.0	3.3
standard	Buitoni	348	13.0	70.0	1.8	3.4
verdi	Buitoni	342	13.4	68.0	1.8	3.5
Lasagne Bolognese Ready Meal	Dolmio	132	7.0	11.7	6.3	n/a
Lasagne Creamy Pasta Bake	Napolina	85.0	2.9	9.4	4.0	0.1
Lasagne Pasta Mix	Colman's	293	8.6	60.0	1.1	n/a
Lasagne Vegetale Ready Meal	Dolmio	101	3.0	11.6	4.7	n/a
Lavash	International Harvest	281	10.4	56.3	1.6	5.5
Lean Cuisine (Findus): ***see individual flavours***						
Lean Roast Beef & Gravy, per pack	Birds Eye	110	15.0	3.4	4.0	0.1

Leek & Potato Cup-A-Soup, per sachet	Batchelors	121	1.5	17.7	4.9	0.5
Leek & Potato Slim-A-Soup, per sachet	Batchelors	56	1.0	10.1	1.4	0.8
Leeks, boiled		21	1.2	2.6	0.7	1.7
Leicester Cheese		401	24.3	0.1	33.7	nil
Lemonade, bottled		21.0	Tr	5.6	nil	nil
	Barr	30.0	n/a	7.4	Tr	Tr
	Corona	10.0	Tr	2.3	nil	n/a
	R Whites	22.5	nil	5.4	Tr	n/a
low calorie	Barr	0.9	n/a	Tr	Tr	Tr
	Corona	1.0	Tr	nil	n/a	n/a
	R Whites	1.4	Tr	Tr	Tr	n/a
Lemon & Dill Marinade	Lea & Perrins	122	0.5	19.1	4.3	n/a
Lemon & Ginger Sauce & Vegetables Stir Fry	Uncle Ben's	61.0	0.6	13.0	0.6	n/a
Lemon & Herb Cod Steaks, each	Birds Eye	195	11.0	16.0	9.8	0.8

All amounts given per 100g/100ml unless otherwise stated

Product	*Brand*	*Calories kcal*	*Protein (g)*	*Carbo-hydrate (g)*	*Fat (g)*	*Dietary Fibre (g)*
Lemon & Lime Crush, per pack	Boots Shapers	7.0	n/a	n/a	Tr	n/a
Lemon & Lime Dessert Mousse	St Ivel Shape	56.0	3.8	4.1	2.3	nil
Lemon & Lime Drink	Jusoda	28.0	n/a	6.9	Tr	Tr
Lemon & Lime Layered Dessert, per pack	Boots Shapers	83.0	n/a	n/a	2.6	n/a
Lemon & Lime Yogurt Mousse	Boots Shapers	93.0	n/a	n/a	3.2	n/a
Lemon Barley Water	Robinsons	88.0	0.3	19.6	Tr	n/a
Lemon Bonbons	Trebor Bassett	417	1.1	85.4	7.5	nil
Lemon Cheesecake Mix	Green's	298	4.0	34.5	16.0	n/a
Lemon Chicken	Findus Lean Cuisine	120	5.5	19.7	1.7	0.8
Lemon Chicken Stir Fry Mix, as sold	Cross & Blackwell	350	3.5	75.2	4.0	nil

Lemon Crunch	Jacob's Vitalinea	415	5.5	76.0	8.0	1.5
Lemon Curd Starch Base		283	0.6	62.7	5.1	0.2
Lemon Curd Tarts	Lyons Cakes	394	3.7	59.2	15.9	n/a
Lemon Delight	Boots Shapers	92.0	n/a	n/a	3.1	n/a
Lemon Dream Bio Yogurt	St Ivel	73.0	5.1	9.7	1.1	Tr
Lemon Drink	Tango	40.0	Tr	9.3	Tr	n/a
low calorie	Tango	3.0	Tr	0.1	Tr	n/a
	Robinsons	11.2	0.2	0.5	Tr	n/a
sparkling	St Clements	47.0	Tr	11.3	Tr	Tr
Lemon Energy Tablets	Lucozade Sport	360	nil	88.8	nil	n/a
Lemon Flavour Jelly Crystals	Dietade	7.0	1.5	0.1	nil	nil
Lemon Hot Crunch Pudding Mix	Bird's	445	5.5	74.0	14.0	0.7
Lemon Iced Slices	Lyons Cakes	377	3.8	58.6	13.2	n/a
Lemon Juice, fresh		7.0	0.3	1.6	Tr	0.1

All amounts given per 100g/100ml unless otherwise stated

Product	*Brand*	*Calories kcal*	*Protein (g)*	*Carbo-hydrate (g)*	*Fat (g)*	*Dietary Fibre (g)*
Lemon Juice Drink	Citrus Spring	41.0	Tr	10.0	Tr	n/a
Lemon Low Calorie Squash	Dietade	7.0	nil	0.4	nil	n/a
Lemon Meringue Crunch Mix	Green's	249	2.5	39.0	9.0	n/a
Lemon Meringue Gateau	McVitie's	276	4.5	25.8	17.9	Tr
Lemon Meringue Pie, recipe		319	4.5	45.9	14.4	0.7
Lemon Pepper Chicken	Birds Eye	242	15.4	17.5	12.3	0.6
Lemon Puff	Jacob's	511	4.5	57.1	29.4	1.6
Lemon Rice	Sharwood	358	7.5	71.9	3.2	1.3
Lemon Sauce, Straight to Wok	Amoy	162	0.1	40.0	0.2	n/a
Lemons, whole, without pips		19.0	1.0	3.2	0.3	N
Lemon Slices	Mr Kipling	395	3.7	58.1	16.1	n/a
Lemon Sole fried in crumbs		216	16.1	9.3	13.0	0.4

steamed		91.0	20.6	nil	0.9	nil
Lemon Sorbet		131	0.9	34.2	Tr	nil
	Del Monte	114	0.1	29.2	Tr	n/a
	Fiesta	114	nil	28.1	nil	n/a
Lemon Sponge Pudding	Heinz	306	2.7	50.1	10.6	0.6
Lemon Whole Fruit Drink	Robinsons	49.0	0.2	9.9	Tr	n/a
Lentil & Bacon Cup-A-Soup, per sachet	Batchelors	89.0	3.4	17.2	0.8	1.2
Lentil & Bacon Soup	Baxters	60.0	2.7	7.9	1.9	0.8
Lentil & Vegetable Soup	Baxters	34.0	1.9	6.8	0.1	1.5
Lentils						
green/brown, boiled		105	8.8	16.9	0.7	3.8
red, boiled		100	7.6	17.5	0.4	1.9
Lentil Soup		99.0	4.4	12.7	3.8	1.1
	Campbell's	27.0	1.3	4.3	0.6	n/a
	Heinz	39.0	2.3	7.1	0.2	1.0

All amounts given per 100g/100ml unless otherwise stated

Product	*Brand*	*Calories kcal*	*Protein (g)*	*Carbo-hydrate (g)*	*Fat (g)*	*Dietary Fibre (g)*
Lerida Figs	Holland & Barrett	240	3.6	52.8	1.6	7.5
Lettuce, average, raw		14.0	0.8	1.7	0.5	0.9
Light & Moist Carrot Cake	California Cake & Cookie Ltd	270	3.1	53.4	3.4	2.7
Light & Moist Chocolate Cake	California Cake & Cookie Ltd	274	4.6	53.1	3.5	3.2
Light & Moist Lemon Cake	California Cake & Cookie Ltd	299	4.3	57.9	3.6	1.9
Light Brown Soft Sugar	Tate & Lyle	384	0.1	95.8	nil	nil
Lightly Salted Crisps	Boots Shapers	482	n/a	n/a	24.0	n/a
Lightly Salted Golden Lights, per pack	Golden Wonder	95.0	1.1	13.8	3.9	0.8
Light Philadelphia Chive & Onion Dip & Breadsticks Handisnack, each	Kraft	117	4.2	12.5	5.7	0.6

Light Philadelphia Dip & Breadsticks Handisnack, each	Kraft	119	4.3	12.0	5.9	0.6
Light Mayonnaise	Hellmanns	299	0.7	6.6	29.8	0.1
Light Soy Chinese Pouring Sauce	Sharwood	18.0	4.4	0.2	Tr	0.3
Lima Beans: ***see Butter Beans***						
Limeade, bottles	Corona	1.3	Tr	n/a	nil	n/a
Lime Cordial,undiluted	Roses	105	0.1	24.4	nil	n/a
Lime Crusha	Burgess	95	nil	22.0	nil	nil
Lime Juice Cordial, undiluted		112	Tr	27.0	nil	nil
	Britvic	46.0	0.1	9.0	Tr	n/a
Lime Juice Drink	Citrus Spring	45.0	Tr	10.6	Tr	n/a
Lime Pickle	Sharwood	152	2.6	2.1	3.6	3.3
Lincoln Biscuits	McVitie's	508	5.8	67.1	23.5	2.0
Lion Bar	Nestlé Rowntree	482	5.0	66.7	21.7	n/a

All amounts given per 100g/100ml unless otherwise stated

Product	Brand	Calories kcal	Protein (g)	Carbo-hydrate (g)	Fat (g)	Dietary Fibre (g)
Lip Smacker, each	Lyons Maid	77.0	nil	19.4	nil	n/a
Liquorice Allsorts		313	3.9	74.1	2.2	N
Liquorice Toffees	Itona	395	0.6	66.5	15.2	n/a
Liquorice Torpedoes	Trebor Bassett	370	3.5	88.3	0.4	1.1
Liver						
calf, fried		254	26.9	7.3	13.2	0.2
chicken, fried		194	20.7	3.4	10.9	0.2
lamb, fried		232	22.9	3.9	14.0	0.1
ox, stewed		198	24.8	3.6	9.5	Tr
pig, stewed		189	25.6	3.6	8.1	Tr
Liver & Bacon Casserole Cooking Mix, as sold	Colman's	289	9.3	59.0	1.2	n/a
Liver Pâté		316	13.1	1.0	28.9	Tr
low fat		191	18.0	2.8	12.0	Tr
Liver Sausage		310	12.9	4.3	26.9	0.5

Lobster, boiled		119	22.1	nil	3.4	nil
	Young's	119	22.1	nil	3.4	nil
Lobster Bisque	Baxters	53.0	3.4	5.2	2.1	0.1
Lockets	Mars	383	nil	95.8	nil	n/a
Lombardy Port Regional Recipe	Ragu	32.0	0.6	7.0	0.2	0.7
Long Grain & Wild Rice, as sold	Uncle Ben's	347	11.2	92.8	1.2	n/a
Long Grain Rice, as sold	Uncle Ben's	342	7.8	75.4	1.0	n/a
	Whitworths	361	6.5	86.8	1.0	0.5
frozen	Uncle Ben's	140	3.0	30.3	0.7	n/a
3 min	Uncle Ben's	127	2.7	27.3	0.8	n/a
Low Fat Dressing	Heinz Weight Watchers	107	1.4	16.0	4.2	nil
Low Fat Spread		390	5.8	0.5	40.5	nil
Lucozade	SmithKline Beecham	73.0	Tr	17.9	nil	nil

All amounts given per 100g/100ml unless otherwise stated

Product	*Brand*	*Calories kcal*	*Protein (g)*	*Carbo-hydrate (g)*	*Fat (g)*	*Dietary Fibre (g)*
Lucozade Orange Crush	SmithKline Beecham	70.0	Tr	17.2	nil	nil
low calorie		5.0	Tr	0.7	nil	nil
Luncheon Meat, canned		313	12.6	5.5	26.9	0.3
Lunchpack & Brussels Pâté, per pack	Boots Shapers	202	n/a	n/a	8.8	n/a
Lunchpack & Cheese, per pack	Boots Shapers	148	n/a	n/a	2.7	n/a
Lunchpack & Cheese & Onion, per pack	Boots Shapers	149	n/a	n/a	2.7	n/a
Lunchpack & Provençal Pâté, per pack	Boots Shapers	198	n/a	n/a	8.0	n/a
Lunchpack with Cheese Spread & Crispbread Scoops, per pack	Boots Shapers	136	n/a	n/a	2.7	n/a

Lunchpack with Dip & Mini Snacks, per pack	Boots Shapers	254	n/a	n/a	13.8	n/a
Luxury Brownies	California Cake & Cookie Ltd	456	5.4	56.7	23.1	0.9
Luxury Mince Pies	Mr Kipling	374	4.0	55.9	14.9	n/a
Luxury Muesli	Jordans	384	9.6	58.4	12.5	8.2
Lychees						
raw		58.0	0.9	14.3	0.1	0.7
canned in syrup		68.0	0.4	17.7	Tr	0.5
	Libby	74.0	n/a	n/a	Tr	n/a

All amounts given per 100g/100ml unless otherwise stated

M

Product	*Brand*	*Calories kcal*	*Protein (g)*	*Carbo-hydrate (g)*	*Fat (g)*	*Dietary Fibre (g)*
M & M's Ice Cream Cone	Mars	319	4.2	36.4	17.4	n/a
Macadamia Nuts, salted		748	7.9	4.8	77.6	5.3
Macaroni, boiled		86.0	3.0	18.5	0.5	0.9
Macaroni Cheese		178	7.3	13.6	10.8	0.5
	Findus Red Box	160	7.0	13.9	8.5	0.7
	Heinz	95.0	3.4	9.8	4.7	0.3
	Birds Eye	124	4.2	15.6	5.0	0.4
Macaroni Cheese Pasta 'n' Sauce	Batchelors	378	17.2	63.6	6.1	2.8

All amounts given per 100g/100ml unless otherwise stated

Product	*Brand*	*Calories kcal*	*Protein (g)*	*Carbo-hydrate (g)*	*Fat (g)*	*Dietary Fibre (g)*
Macaroni with Chicken & Bacon	Findus	145	5.5	14.2	7.4	0.7
Macaroni with Ham & Leek, as sold	Findus	140	4.5	15.5	6.6	0.8
McChicken Sandwich, each	McDonald's	375	16.5	38.5	17.2	3.8
Mackerel, fried, flesh only		188	21.5	nil	11.3	nil
Madeira Cake		393	5.4	58.4	16.9	0.9
Madeira Loaf Mix	Green's	339	4.9	56.0	12.4	n/a
Madeira Wine Gravy Sauce Dry Mix, as sold	Crosse & Blackwell	355	8.4	59.1	7.2	1.2
Madras Classic Curry Sauce	Homepride	67.0	1.9	13.3	0.8	n/a
Madras Curry Sauce	Sharwood	100	1.7	6.9	7.3	1.6
Major Grey Chutney	Sharwood	215	0.4	52.9	0.2	1.0

Malaysian Chicken & Sweetcorn Soups of the World	Knorr	387	11.1	59.6	11.6	1.9
Malaysian Mild Curry Paste	Sharwood	252	5.2	9.9	21.1	6.6
Malt Bread		268	8.3	56.8	2.4	N
Malted Food Drink (Horlicks): ***see Horlicks***						
Maltesers	Mars	494	10.0	61.4	23.1	n/a
Malt Extract	Holland & Barrett	300	0.4	78.0	nil	nil
Maltissimo Low Fat Milk Chocolate Drink	SmithKline Beecham	394	14.6	62.4	9.6	6.8
Maltissimo Low Fat Mocha Flavoured Chocolate Drink	SmithKline Beecham	65.0	2.2	10.6	1.5	1.5
Maltissimo Low Fat Tiramisu Flavoured Drink	SmithKline Beecham	65.0	2.3	10.6	1.5	1.5
Mandarin Chocolate Cake	Lyons Cakes	412	5.1	48.8	20.5	n/a
Mandarin Chocolate Roll	Lyons Cakes	380	4.4	53.1	15.4	n/a

All amounts given per 100g/100ml unless otherwise stated

Product	Brand	Calories kcal	Protein (g)	Carbo-hydrate (g)	Fat (g)	Dietary Fibre (g)
Mandarin Delight, per pack	Boots Shapers	120	n/a	n/a	4.8	n/a
Mandarin Oranges						
canned in juice		32.0	0.7	7.7	Tr	0.3
	Libby	41.0	n/a	n/a	Tr	n/a
canned in syrup		52.0	0.5	14.4	Tr	0.2
	Libby	57.0	n/a	n/a	Tr	n/a
Mange-tout, raw		32.0	3.6	4.2	0.2	2.3
boiled		26.0	3.2	3.3	0.1	2.2
stir-fried		71.0	3.8	3.5	4.8	2.4
Mango & Apple Chutney	Sharwood	233	0.4	57.6	0.1	1.1
Mango & Chilli Pickle	Sharwood	83.0	2.0	3.4	5.9	3.4
Mango & Lime Chutney	Sharwood	206	0.4	50.5	0.3	0.8
Mango Chutney, oily		285	0.4	49.5	10.9	0.9
Mango Chutney	Sharwood Green Label	234	0.3	57.8	0.2	0.9
	Burgess	279	0.2	61.0	3.1	0.8

Mangoes						
ripe, raw, flesh only		57.0	0.7	14.1	0.2	2.6
canned in syrup		77.0	0.3	20.3	Tr	0.7
	Libby	70.0	n/a	n/a	Tr	n/a
Mango Fromage Frais	St Ivel Shape	70.0	6.9	7.2	1.2	Tr
Mango Sorbet	Del Monte	115	0.2	29.6	Tr	n/a
Mango with Ginger Chutney	Baxters	187	0.5	45.7	0.2	0.9
Manor House Cake	Mr Kipling	423	5.2	53.5	20.9	n/a
Maple & Pecan Crunchy Bar, each	Jordans	155	2.6	18.9	7.6	2.2
Maple & Pecan Original Crunchy	Jordans	448	9.9	59.9	18.7	6.5
Maple Syrup Pancakes	Sunblest	268	5.1	54.2	3.4	0.9
Maple Walnut Cake	California Cake & Cookie Ltd	470	4.1	59.3	24.0	0.7
Maple Walnut Napoli	Lyons Maid	118	2.0	12.9	6.5	n/a
Margarine, average		739	0.2	1.0	81.6	nil

All amounts given per 100g/100ml unless otherwise stated

Product	*Brand*	*Calories kcal*	*Protein (g)*	*Carbo-hydrate (g)*	*Fat (g)*	*Dietary Fibre (g)*
Marble	Cadbury	535	8.4	54.8	31.2	n/a
Marble Choc & Vanilla Slice	Mr Kipling	458	3.5	50.6	24.6	n/a
Marmalade		261	0.1	69.5	nil	0.6
sucrose free	Dietade	267	0.2	66.4	Tr	nil
Marmite		172	39.7	1.8	0.7	nil
Marmite Stock Cubes	Bestfoods	247	25.0	25.5	5.0	n/a
Marmite Yeast Extract	Bestfoods	208	45.0	7.0	Tr	4.0
Marrow						
raw, flesh only		12.0	0.5	2.2	0.2	0.5
boiled		9.0	0.4	1.6	0.2	0.6
Marrowfat Peas, canned		100	6.9	17.5	0.8	4.1
Mars Bar	Mars	452	4.0	69.6	17.5	n/a
Dark Ice Cream	Mars	349	3.7	37.5	20.5	n/a
Ice Cream Bar	Mars	346	5.1	37.2	19.7	n/a
Marzipan, homemade		461	10.4	50.2	25.8	3.3
retail		404	5.3	67.6	14.4	1.9

Matchmakers: ***see individual flavours***						
Mature Cheese, reduced fat	Heinz Weight Watchers	306	27.0	0.1	22.0	nil
Matzo Crackers	Rakusen	335	10.8	76.7	0.4	5.7
Maverick	Nestlé Rowntree	467	4.1	63.4	21.9	0.9
Maxibon	Nestlé	209	2.4	23.4	11.7	n/a
Maya Gold Chocolate, organic	Green & Black's	556	7.5	53.1	34.8	nil
Mayonnaise		691	1.1	1.7	75.6	nil
	Heinz	734	1.5	0.4	80.7	nil
light	Heinz Weight Watchers	131	1.6	9.7	9.5	nil
Meatfree Ravioli in Tomato Sauce	Heinz	75.0	2.4	14.4	0.8	0.5
Meatfree Spaghetti Bolognese	Heinz	86.0	3.1	13.1	2.4	0.7
Meat Paste		173	15.2	3.0	11.2	0.1

All amounts given per 100g/100ml unless otherwise stated

Product	Brand	Calories kcal	Protein (g)	Carbo-hydrate (g)	Fat (g)	Dietary Fibre (g)
Mediterranean Chutney	Baxters	119	1.8	26.0	0.9	1.3
Mediterranean Make a Meal	Birds Eye	57.0	3.3	5.9	2.2	1.3
Mediterranean Tomato & Vegetable Soup	Heinz Weight Watchers	18.0	0.6	3.3	0.3	0.4
Mediterranean Tomato Slim-A-Soup, per sachet	Batchelors	54.0	1.1	9.7	1.2	0.9
Mediterranean Tomato Soup	Baxters	30.0	1.1	6.3	0.3	0.6
	Campbell's	28.0	0.6	6.4	Tr	n/a
Mediterranean Tuna Pocket with Mixed Leaf, per pack	Boots Shapers	294	19.0	37.0	7.8	5.0
Medium Curry Paste	Sharwood	369	4.3	14.0	32.8	6.9
Medium Egg Noodles	Amoy	169	6.0	24.5	5.2	n/a
	Sharwood	340	10.8	70.1	1.8	2.9
Medium Fat Soft Cheese		179	9.2	3.1	14.5	nil
Mega King Cone, each	Lyons Maid	367	6.2	46.4	18.7	n/a

Mega Mint King Cone, each	Lyons Maid	367	6.2	46.4	18.7	n/a
Mega Truffle	Nestlé	289	3.7	26.0	19.0	n/a
Mello Spread	St Ivel	510	0.2	1.3	56.0	nil
Melon, flesh only						
Cantaloupe-type		19.0	0.6	4.2	0.1	1.0
Galia		24.0	0.5	5.6	0.1	0.4
Honeydew		28.0	0.6	6.6	0.1	0.6
Watermelon		31.0	0.5	7.1	0.3	0.1
Meringue		379	5.3	95.4	Tr	nil
Mexican Chilli Cooking Sauce	Heinz Weight Watchers	37.0	1.5	7.0	0.3	1.2
Mexican Chilli with Deep Fried Potato Wedges	Heinz Weight Watchers	84.0	5.1	10.3	2.5	1.7
Mexican Griddlers, each	Birds Eye	180	12.0	5.6	12.0	0.4
Mexican Hot Chilli Sauce	Homepride	40.0	1.3	8.2	0.2	n/a
Mexican Medium Chilli Sauce	Homepride	41.0	1.4	8.7	0.1	n/a

Product	*Brand*	*Calories kcal*	*Protein (g)*	*Carbo-hydrate (g)*	*Fat (g)*	*Dietary Fibre (g)*
Mexican Herb & Spice Cubes, each	Oxo	16.0	0.8	2.4	0.4	0.2
Mickey, each	Lyons Maid	98.0	2.2	11.7	4.7	n/a
Micro Chips	McCain	193	2.5	27.4	8.2	n/a
Midnight Hot Chocolate, per pack	Boots Shapers	40.0	n/a	n/a	0.9	n/a
Mighty White Bread	Allied Bakeries	224	7.2	45.5	1.5	3.7
Milanese Chicken Regional Recipe	Ragu	48.8	0.9	4.9	2.9	0.9
Mild Beer: ***see Beer***						
Mild Cheese & Broccoli Pasta 'n' Sauce	Batchelors	371	13.5	69.0	4.5	2.8
Mild Cheese, reduced fat	Heinz Weight Watchers	306	27.0	0.1	22.0	nil
Mild Chilli Seasoning Dry Sauce Mix, as sold	Colman's	322	9.2	60.0	3.9	n/a

Mild Curry Beanfeast, per packet, as served	Batchelors	328	21.1	44.1	7.5	12.5
Mild Curry Paste	Sharwood	356	4.8	4.8	35.3	7.1
Mild Curry Savoury Rice	Batchelors	355	8.4	76.0	1.9	1.8
Mild Curry Supernoodles	Batchelors	480	10.0	63.6	20.7	3.2
Mild Mustard Low Fat Dressing	Heinz Weight Watchers	63.0	2.0	5.7	3.6	nil
Mild Mustard Pickle	Heinz Speciality	128	2.4	26.7	1.3	1.0
Mild Vegetable Curry	Sharwood	66.0	1.5	4.9	4.5	1.0
Milk (see also condensed, soya, etc.)						
semi-skimmed, average		46.0	3.3	5.0	1.6	nil
skimmed, average		33.0	3.3	5.0	0.1	nil
whole, average		66.0	3.2	4.8	3.9	nil
Milk & Plain Chocolate Caramels	Cravens	493	Tr	96.4	nil	nil
Milk Chocolate		529	8.4	59.4	30.3	Tr
organic	Green & Black's	541	9.3	56.0	31.0	nil

All amounts given per 100g/100ml unless otherwise stated

Product	*Brand*	*Calories kcal*	*Protein (g)*	*Carbo-hydrate (g)*	*Fat (g)*	*Dietary Fibre (g)*
Milk Chocolate Aero	Nestlé Rowntree	518	7.6	57.2	28.8	0.9
Milk Chocolate Breakaway	Nestlé Rowntree	498	6.6	59.1	26.1	n/a
Milk Chocolate Club Biscuits	Jacob's	514	5.5	60.8	27.6	2.5
Milk Chocolate Flavour Custard Dessert	Ambrosia	120	2.9	21.0	2.7	0.8
Milk Chocolate Finger Biscuits	Cadbury	526	6.9	64.3	26.8	1.8
Milk Chocolate Mousse, per pack	Boots Shapers	88.0	n/a	n/a	2.8	n/a
Milk Chocolate Multipack, per pack	Boots Shapers	198	n/a	n/a	4.5	n/a
Milk Chocolate Yorkie	Nestlé Rowntree	526	6.5	58.5	29.5	n/a
Milk Classico, each	Lyons Maid	141	1.7	13.5	9.0	n/a
Milk Jestives	Cadbury	506	6.5	65.4	24.3	2.4

Milk Pudding						
made with whole milk		129	3.9	19.9	4.3	0.1
made with semi-skimmed milk		93.0	4.0	20.1	0.2	0.1
Milk Stick, each	Nestlé	275	3.5	23.6	18.5	n/a
Milk Tray	Cadbury	505	5.6	60.5	26.6	n/a
Milky Bar/Buttons	Nestlé Rowntree	542	7.6	57.5	31.3	nil
Milky Bar Fromage Frais	Chambourcy	215	4.4	23.3	11.3	nil
Milkybar Ice Cream, each	Nestlé	114	2.0	9.6	7.5	n/a
Milky Bar Melted Dessert	Chambourcy	250	4.7	21.7	16.1	nil
Milky Way	Mars	454	4.2	72.0	16.6	n/a
Milky Way Ice Cream Bar	Mars	348	4.8	31.5	22.5	n/a
Milky Way Magic Stars	Mars	564	8.5	51.5	36.0	n/a
Mince & Tomato Casserole Mix, as sold	Colman's	309	9.7	63.0	0.9	n/a
Mince, Beans & Barbecue Sauce	Tyne Brand	109	8.1	11.6	3.4	n/a

All amounts given per 100g/100ml unless otherwise stated

Product	*Brand*	*Calories kcal*	*Protein (g)*	*Carbo-hydrate (g)*	*Fat (g)*	*Dietary Fibre (g)*
Mince Bolognese	Tyne Brand	116	10.2	4.7	6.3	n/a
Minced Beef: *see Beef*						
Minced Beef & Onion	Tyne Brand	115	9.5	7.0	5.5	n/a
Minced Beef & Onion Deep Pie	Ross	249	6.0	24.6	14.5	1.0
Minced Beef & Onion Pie	Ross	295	6.6	24.6	19.4	1.0
	Tyne Brand	161	8.7	13.3	8.1	n/a
Minced Beef Crispy Pancakes	Findus	170	6.1	22.8	5.8	0.9
Minced Beef with Vegetables & Gravy, per pack	Birds Eye	155	16.0	9.0	6.0	1.0
Mincemeat		274	0.6	62.1	4.3	1.3
Mince, Pasta & Tomato Sauce	Tyne Brand	117	7.8	9.3	5.4	n/a
Mince Pies	Mr Kipling	379	3.8	59.0	14.2	n/a
Mince Slices	Mr Kipling	379	3.5	58.9	14.3	n/a

Minestrone Cup-A-Soup, per sachet	Batchelors	100	1.9	17.9	2.3	1.1
Minestrone Soup	Knorr	283	10.3	52.7	3.4	7.7
Minestrone Packet Soup	Batchelors	26	0.7	5.1	0.3	0.4
Minestrone Slim-A-Soup, per sachet	Batchelors	53.0	1.4	9.3	1.3	1.2
Minestrone Soup, canned	Baxters	34.0	1.3	6.0	0.6	0.8
	Heinz	30.0	1.3	4.8	0.6	0.6
	Heinz Weight Watchers	20.0	0.8	3.3	0.4	0.4
Minestrone Soup, dried						
as served		23.0	0.8	3.7	8.8	N
as sold		298	10.1	47.6	8.8	N
Minestrone with Pasta Cup-A-Soup Extra, per sachet	Batchelors	123	3.9	24.3	1.1	2.3
Minestrone with Wholemeal Pasta	Baxters	32.0	0.9	6.7	0.2	1.0

All amounts given per 100g/100ml unless otherwise stated

Product	*Brand*	*Calories kcal*	*Protein (g)*	*Carbo-hydrate (g)*	*Fat (g)*	*Dietary Fibre (g)*
Mini Crispbread, per pack	Boots Shapers	68.0	n/a	n/a	0.5	n/a
Mini Muesli Crispbreads, per pack	Boots Shapers	84.0	n/a	n/a	0.9	n/a
Mini Pizza Bases	Napolina	298	8.5	56.0	4.4	n/a
Mini Yum Yums	Sunblest	397	5.3	52.5	18.4	1.3
Mint Aero	Nestlé Rowntree	518	7.6	57.2	28.8	0.9
Mint Assortment	Cravens	414	0.3	89.4	6.1	nil
Mint Choc Chip King Cone, each	Lyons Maid	185	3.0	23.6	8.6	n/a
Mint Choc Chip Mousse, each	Fiesta	84.0	1.8	10.6	4.1	n/a
Mint Choc Chip Napoli	Lyons Maid	124	2.1	13.7	6.8	n/a
Mint Chocolate, organic	Green & Black's	541	9.3	56.0	31.0	nil
Mint Club Biscuits	Jacob's	520	5.0	62.1	27.9	1.9
Mint Crisp	Cadbury	505	6.4	70.3	22.2	n/a

Mint Crisp Chocolates	Elizabeth Shaw	458	1.9	68.0	20.7	1.7
Mint Crisp, each	Lyons Maid	198	1.7	22.0	11.4	n/a
Mint Crisp Trio	Elizabeth Shaw	494	4.4	67.6	22.9	0.7
Mint Duo de Mousse Dessert	Chambourcy	185	4.3	18.3	10.6	0.1
Minted Garden Peas	Ross	72.0	6.0	14.5	0.8	4.3
Mintetts	G. Payne & Co	395	Tr	92.7	27.0	n/a
Mint Humbugs	Cravens	413	0.6	89.7	5.8	nil
Mint Imperials	Cravens	387	nil	96.3	nil	nil
	Trebor Bassett	396	0.4	98.1	0.2	nil
Mint Jelly	Baxters	264	nil	66.0	nil	nil
	Burgess	165	0.4	37.6	0.7	0.5
	Colman's	249	0.2	61.0	Tr	n/a
Mint Matchmakers	Nestlé Rowntree	477	5.1	68.7	20.2	n/a
Mint Munchies	Nestlé Rowntree	433	3.8	67.4	16.5	n/a
Mints: ***see individual types***						

All amounts given per 100g/100ml unless otherwise stated

Product	*Brand*	*Calories kcal*	*Protein (g)*	*Carbo-hydrate (g)*	*Fat (g)*	*Dietary Fibre (g)*
Mint Sauce	Baxters	62.0	1.7	13.2	0.3	nil
	Burgess	68	1.6	12.0	nil	2.0
	Colman's	122	0.8	26.0	0.1	n/a
Mint Toffees	Itona	360	0.6	67.0	11.0	n/a
Mint YoYo	McVitie's	523	4.7	63.9	27.7	0.8
Minty Chews	Trebor Bassett	395	0.8	84.2	6.1	nil
Miracle Whip Dressing	Kraft	400	0.3	11.0	39.0	0.1
Miso		203	13.3	23.5	6.2	N
Mississippi Mud Pie	Green's	323	4.0	37.5	17.5	n/a
Mivvis (Lyons Maid): ***see individual flavours***						
Mixed Fruit, dried		227	3.6	52.9	1.6	2.2
Mixed Fruit Sponge Pudding	Heinz	302	4.0	44.5	12.0	1.3
Mixed Fruit Sucrose Free Jam	Dietade	245	0.3	60.3	Tr	n/a

Mixed Herbs Cubes	Knorr	464	5.4	35.3	33.5	0.8
Mixed Nuts		607	22.9	7.9	54.1	6.0
Mixed Peel		231	0.3	59.1	0.9	4.8
Mixed Peppers, dried	Whitworths	212	21.7	21.7	4.9	8.9
Mixed Vegetables						
frozen, boiled		42.0	3.3	6.6	0.5	N
canned		38.0	1.9	6.1	0.8	1.7
stir fry type, frozen, fried in oil		64.0	2.0	6.4	3.6	N
Mocha Hot Chocolate, per pack	Boots Shapers	40.0	n/a	n/a	0.9	n/a
Moghlai Chicken Korma Microwave Meal	Sharwood	162	7.0	17.0	7.8	1.4
Monkey Nuts: ***see Peanuts***						
Montego Lemon	Nestlé	105	1.0	20.6	2.1	n/a
Montego Orange	Nestlé	110	0.6	21.6	2.3	n/a
Montego Raspberry	Nestlé	103	0.6	21.8	1.6	n/a
Mooli: ***see Radish, white***						

Product	*Brand*	*Calories kcal*	*Protein (g)*	*Carbo-hydrate (g)*	*Fat (g)*	*Dietary Fibre (g)*
Moonshine	Libby	48.0	Tr	12.0	Tr	nil
Moussaka		184	9.1	7.0	13.6	0.9
Mousse: *see individual flavours*						
Mr Brain's Faggots in West Country Sauce	Hibernia Brands	131	7.2	11.7	6.2	0.3
Mrs Peek's Rum & Brandy Pudding	Jacob's	335	2.9	34.9	7.1	4.5
Mrs Peek's Cider & Sherry Pudding	Jacob's	326	2.6	60.7	8.1	3.1
Muesli						
Swiss style		363	9.8	72.2	5.9	6.4
with no added sugar		366	10.5	67.1	7.8	7.6
Muffins	Sunblest	240	8.8	47.6	1.6	2.0
Mulligatawny Beef Curry Soup	Heinz	60.0	1.8	7.2	2.7	0.5

Multi Cheerios	Nestlé	369	7.9	75.9	3.8	6.2
Multiflake	Doves Farm	354	11.8	69.5	3.2	7.9
Multigrain Ryvita, per slice	Ryvita	37.0	1.3	6.4	0.7	1.8
Multi-Grain Start	Kellogg's	360	8.0	79.0	2.0	6.0
Munchies	Nestlé Rowntree	488	5.1	62.5	24.2	0.6
Munchies Dessert Split Pot	Chambourcy	245	4.4	30.0	12.0	n/a
Munchmallows	McVitie's	448	5.3	70.0	16.5	1.1
Mung beans, boiled		91.0	7.6	15.3	0.4	4.8
Mung Beansprouts: *see Beansprouts*						
Murray Mints	Trebor Bassett	409	nil	90.3	5.3	nil
Mushroom & Bacon Toast Topper	Heinz	94.0	6.9	6.6	4.4	0.3
Mushroom & Cheese filled Pasta, as sold	Findus	100	3.0	13.7	3.9	0.5

All amounts given per 100g/100ml unless otherwise stated

Product	*Brand*	*Calories kcal*	*Protein (g)*	*Carbo-hydrate (g)*	*Fat (g)*	*Dietary Fibre (g)*
Mushroom & Cheese with Bacon & Croutons Cup-A-Soup	Batchelors	129	1.7	16.8	6.1	0.5
Mushroom & Garlic Low In Fat Sauce	Homepride	51.0	1.1	8.9	1.4	n/a
Mushroom & Garlic Pizza	San Marco	241	11.3	28.5	10.4	1.2
Mushroom & Garlic with White Wine Soup	Campbell's	53.0	0.7	3.8	3.9	n/a
Mushroom & Pepper Soup	Campbell's	42.0	0.4	3.3	3.0	n/a
Mushroom & Wine Pasta 'n' Sauce	Batchelors	377	12.0	71.3	4.9	2.5
Mushroom Ketchup	Burgess	27.0	0.5	5.5	0.1	Tr
Mushroom Parisienne Bake	Birds Eye	92.0	9.8	2.9	4.6	0.2
Mushroom Pasta Sauce	Dolmio	36.0	0.9	8.2	Tr	n/a

Mushroom Pâté	Tartex	235	7.0	9.0	18.5	n/a
per tub	Vessen	120	2.9	5.8	9.4	0.1
Mushroom Sauce	Ragu	68.0	2.0	9.5	2.1	1.2
Mushrooms						
common, raw		13.0	1.8	0.4	0.5	1.1
common, boiled		11.0	1.8	0.4	0.3	1.1
common, fried in oil		157	2.4	0.3	16.2	1.5
common, canned		12.0	2.1	Tr	0.4	1.3
Chinese, dried, raw		284	10.0	59.9	1.8	N
oyster, raw		8.0	1.6	Tr	0.2	N
shiitake, dried, raw		296	9.6	63.9	1.0	N
shiitake, cooked		55.0	1.6	12.3	0.2	N
straw, canned, drained		15.0	2.1	1.2	0.2	N
Mushroom Sauce Mix, as sold	Colman's	358	14.0	53.0	9.7	n/a
Mushroom Savoury Rice	Batchelors	360	10.9	74.3	2.1	2.5
Mushroom Soup	Heinz Weight Watchers	32.0	1.3	5.0	0.7	0.1

All amounts given per 100g/100ml unless otherwise stated

Product	*Brand*	*Calories kcal*	*Protein (g)*	*Carbo-hydrate (g)*	*Fat (g)*	*Dietary Fibre (g)*
Mushroom Supernoodles	Batchelors	477	9.8	63.5	20.7	3.2
Mushy Mint Peas	Batchelors	74.0	5.7	12.1	4.0	2.6
Mushy Peas, canned		81.0	5.8	13.8	0.7	1.8
	Batchelors	77.0	5.2	13.5	0.2	2.7
Mushy Peas Chip Shop Style	Batchelors	67.0	5.4	15.8	0.4	n/a
Mussels, boiled		87.0	17.2	Tr	2.0	nil
Mustard						
smooth		139	7.1	9.7	8.2	N
wholegrain		140	8.2	4.2	10.2	4.9

N

Product	*Brand*	*Calories kcal*	*Protein (g)*	*Carbo-hydrate (g)*	*Fat (g)*	*Dietary Fibre (g)*
Naan Bread		336	8.9	50.1	12.5	1.9
Nacho Dippits	Primula	336	7.8	18.4	25.7	n/a
Napoletana Pasta Express Sauce	Buitoni	72.0	1.5	6.8	4.2	n/a
Napoletana Pasta Sauce, chilled	Dolmio	49.0	1.3	7.0	1.8	n/a
Napoletana Pasta Sauce with Red Wine & Herbs (jar)	Dolmio	30.0	0.8	6.6	Tr	n/a

All amounts given per 100g/100ml unless otherwise stated

Product	*Brand*	*Calories kcal*	*Protein (g)*	*Carbo-hydrate (g)*	*Fat (g)*	*Dietary Fibre (g)*
Natural Bio Yogurt	Holland & Barrett	54.0	4.4	5.6	1.5	nil
Natural Bran	Jordans	213	14.1	26.8	5.5	36.4
Natural Cod Steaks, each	Birds Eye	70.0	17.0	nil	0.3	nil
Natural Harvest Marrowfat Peas	Batchelors	82.0	5.8	13.8	0.4	0.2
Natural Muesli	Jordans	352	10.4	62.4	6.7	8.9
Natural Wheat Bran	Holland & Barrett	171	12.5	25.0	3.0	43.0
Natural Wheat Germ	Jordans	345	26.5	39.6	9.0	13.7
Natural Yogurt, low fat	St Ivel	64.0	5.6	6.5	1.2	nil
Neapolitan Ice Cream	Fiesta	173	3.6	20.1	9.3	n/a
	Lyons Maid	87.0	1.8	11.0	4.0	n/a
Nectarine & Apricot Yogurt	St Ivel Shape	54.0	5.3	6.8	0.2	0.1

Nectarine & Mango Bio Yogurt	St Ivel Shape	55.0	5.4	6.9	0.2	0.1
Nectarine Bio Stirred Yogurt	Ski	112	5.8	16.7	2.9	nil
Nectarines, flesh & skin		40.0	1.4	9.0	0.1	1.2
Neeps (England): *see Swede*						
Neeps (Scotland): *see Turnip*						
Nescafé Original	Nescafé	100	13.9	10.0	0.1	16.2
Nesquik Breakfast Cereal	Nestlé	382	5.3	84.7	2.5	2.7
Nesquik (Nestlé): *see individual flavours*						
New Potatoes: *see Potatoes, new*						
Niblets	Green Giant	100	2.7	20.8	0.7	1.2
Niblets Extra Crisp	Green Giant	70.0	2.7	13.3	0.7	2.7
Niblets, no salt, no sugar	Green Giant	77.0	2.6	16.7	nil	2.6
Niblets with Peppers	Green Giant	82.0	2.6	17.9	nil	1.3

Product	*Brand*	*Calories kcal*	*Protein (g)*	*Carbo-hydrate (g)*	*Fat (g)*	*Dietary Fibre (g)*
Nice 'n' Spicy Nik Naks, per pack	Golden Wonder	185	1.6	18.9	11.4	0.3
Nice 'n' Spicy Pot Noodle	Golden Wonder	424	11.7	56.4	16.8	3.9
Nice Biscuits	Jacob's	471	6.1	69.0	18.9	1.8
95% Fat Free Creamy Ranch Dressing	Kraft	111	1.4	14.5	5.0	0.3
95% Fat Free Creamy Ranch Dressing with Blue Cheese	Kraft	107	0.8	14.0	5.0	Tr
95% Fat Free Creamy Ranch Dressing with Spring Onion and Chive	Kraft	113	1.3	15.0	5.0	0.4
99% Fat Free Soup	Campbell's					
Chicken		34.0	1.6	5.0	0.9	n/a
Mushroom		24.0	0.6	3.5	0.9	n/a
Spicy Tomato		30.0	0.6	6.9	Tr	n/a
Tomato		44.0	0.7	8.0	1.0	n/a

No Bake Egg Custard Mix	Green's	109	3.5	13.5	4.5	n/a
Nobble	Cadbury	460	4.8	68.6	18.4	n/a
Nobbly Bobbly, each	Lyons Maid	147	1.4	22.0	5.9	n/a
Non-dairy Ice Cream: *see Ice Cream*						
Noodles, egg, boiled		62.0	2.2	13.0	0.5	0.6
Norfolk Chicken Sauce, as sold	Colman's	99	1.2	5.8	7.9	1.0
North Atlantic Peeled Prawns	Young's	61.0	15.1	nil	0.1	nil
Noughts & Crosses	Doves Farm	362	8.5	76.7	2.3	4.0
No. 7 Cider	H P Bulmer	34.0	n/a	n/a	n/a	n/a
Nut Meringue Gateau	McVitie's	407	3.0	32.4	29.5	Tr
Nuts about Caramel	Cadbury	495	5.5	58.1	26.7	n/a
Nutty Oatios	Mornflake	447	9.0	61.0	18.6	4.8

All amounts given per 100g/100ml unless otherwise stated

O

Product	*Brand*	*Calories kcal*	*Protein (g)*	*Carbo-hydrate (g)*	*Fat (g)*	*Dietary Fibre (g)*
Oat & Wheat Bran	Weetabix	334	11.7	60.2	5.2	16.9
Oatbran	Mornflake	348	16.5	52.5	8.0	14.6
Oat Crispy Crunch	Mornflake	434	6.3	68.9	14.3	5.0
Oat Danish Bread	Heinz Weight Watchers	227	10.7	38.6	3.3	7.7
Oat Fingers, each	Paterson's	45.0	n/a	n/a	1.9	n/a
Oat Krunchies	Quaker	393	9.5	72.0	7.0	5.5

All amounts given per 100g/100ml unless otherwise stated

Product	Brand	Calories kcal	Protein (g)	Carbo-hydrate (g)	Fat (g)	Dietary Fibre (g)
Oatcakes		441	10.0	63.0	18.3	N
Oatmeal (Medium, Coarse or Fine)	Mornflake	364	11.8	62.0	7.6	7.2
Oatmeal Bread	Crofters Kitchen	234	8.1	41.6	3.9	3.7
Ocean Pie	Heinz Baked Bean Cuisine	91.0	5.9	10.1	3.0	1.3
	Ross	121	7.0	9.8	6.2	0.4
Ocean Pie with Cod	Heinz Weight Watchers	85.0	5.4	10.0	2.6	0.8
Okra (gumbo, lady's fingers)						
boiled		28.0	2.5	2.7	0.9	3.6
stir-fried		269	4.3	4.4	26.1	6.3
canned, drained		21.0	1.4	2.5	0.7	2.6
Old English Toffee Oatso Simple	Quaker	374	8.0	71.0	6.0	5.0
Old Jamaica	Cadbury	460	5.8	56.9	23.3	n/a

Olive Oil		899	Tr	nil	99.9	nil
Olives, pitted, in brine		103	0.9	Tr	11.0	2.9
Olivio	Van den Bergh	571	0.4	0.7	63.0	nil
Omelette, plain		191	10.9	Tr	16.4	nil
cheese		266	15.9	Tr	22.6	nil
Onion & Chive Dip	Primula	341	4.6	2.1	34.9	n/a
Onion & Garlic 95% Fat Free Dip	St Ivel Shape	83.0	6.7	5.9	3.7	0.1
Onion & Garlic Soured Cream Dip	St Ivel	402	2.2	3.4	42.2	0.3
Onion Bhajia Mix	Sharwood	222	4.8	25.6	11.2	3.6
Onion Bhajis	Ross	151	5.7	25.8	3.9	2.5
Onion Crunchies	Ross	136	2.5	23.4	4.2	1.4
Onion, Garlic & Herb Soured Cream Dip	St Ivel	410	2.2	3.4	43.1	0.2
Onion Granules, as sold	Oxo	328	8.2	62.3	4.8	0.8

All amounts given per 100g/100ml unless otherwise stated

Product	*Brand*	*Calories kcal*	*Protein (g)*	*Carbo-hydrate (g)*	*Fat (g)*	*Dietary Fibre (g)*
Onions						
raw		36.0	1.2	7.9	0.2	1.4
baked		103	3.5	22.3	0.6	3.9
boiled		17.0	0.6	3.7	0.1	0.7
fried in oil		164	2.3	14.1	11.2	3.1
dried, raw		313	10.2	68.6	1.7	12.1
pickled, drained		24.0	0.9	4.9	0.2	1.2
cocktail/silverskin, drained		15.0	0.6	3.1	0.1	N
Onion Sauce						
made with whole milk		99.0	2.8	8.3	6.5	0.4
made with semi-skimmed milk		86.0	2.9	8.4	5.0	0.4
Onion Sauce Mix, as sold	Colman's	316	8.3	68.0	1.0	n/a
	Knorr	383	6.1	42.6	21.0	3.2
Onion Wholegrain Crispbread	Kavli	368	10.0	67.4	6.5	11.3
Orangeade	Corona	1.5	Tr	Tr	nil	n/a
Orange Aero	Nestlé Rowntree	518	7.6	57.2	28.8	0.9

Orange & Lemon Gateau	McVitie's	292	2.4	31.7	17.5	0.4
Orange &Mango Fruit Juice	Del Monte	46.0	0.6	10.4	Tr	n/a
Orange & Mango Special R	Robinsons	35.0	0.2	0.9	Tr	n/a
Orange & Peach C-Vit Ready to Drink	SmithKline Beecham	37.0	Tr	9.0	nil	n/a
Orange & Pineapple Drink						
as sold	Tango	40.0	Tr	9.6	Tr	n/a
	Quosh	55.0	0.1	12.4	Tr	n/a
low calorie	Tango	3.3	Tr	0.5	Tr	n/a
Orange & Pineapple Fruit Juice	Del Monte	48.0	0.5	11.0	Tr	n/a
Orange & Pineapple Special R, as sold	Robinsons	8.2	0.2	0.9	Tr	n/a
Orange & Pineapple Whole Fruit Drink	Robinsons	43.0	0.1	9.6	Tr	n/a
Orange & Raspberry Drink, per 250ml pack	Boots Shapers	111	n/a	n/a	Tr	n/a

All amounts given per 100g/100ml unless otherwise stated

Product	*Brand*	*Calories kcal*	*Protein (g)*	*Carbo-hydrate (g)*	*Fat (g)*	*Dietary Fibre (g)*
Orange Apple Passionfruit Juice	Del Monte	45.0	0.5	10.1	Tr	n/a
Orange Bar, each	Boots Shapers	96.0	n/a	n/a	3.8	n/a
Orange Barley Water	Robinsons	89.0	0.3	21.0	Tr	n/a
Orange 'C'	Libby	37.0	0.1	9.1	Tr	0.1
no added sugar	Libby	12.0	0.2	1.9	Tr	Tr
Orange Chewits	Leaf	392	0.4	90.8	3.0	nil
Orange Club Biscuits	Jacob's	521	5.0	61.8	28.2	1.9
Orange Cream	Cadbury	425	2.6	68.6	15.4	n/a
Orange Crush, per pack	Boots Shapers	22.0	n/a	n/a	Tr	n/a
Orange C-Vit, Ready to Drink	SmithKline Beecham	42.0	Tr	10.1	nil	n/a
Orange Drink	Citrus Spring	41.0	Tr	10.0	Tr	n/a
	Jusoda	31.0	n/a	7.6	Tr	Tr
	Tango	44.0	Tr	10.6	Tr	n/a

undiluted		107	Tr	28.5	nil	nil
	Quosh	40.0	0.1	8.8	Tr	n/a
sparkling	St Clements	47.0	n/a	11.1	Tr	Tr
low calorie	Boots Shapers	2.0	n/a	n/a	Tr	n/a
	Tango	4.7	Tr	0.7	Tr	n/a
Orange Flavour Jelly Crystals	Dietade	7.0	1.5	0.1	nil	nil
Orange Fruit Burst	Del Monte	49.0	0.1	12.0	Tr	n/a
Orange Fruit Juice	Del Monte	44.0	0.6	9.9	Tr	n/a
Orange Energy Tablets	Lucozade Sport	361	nil	88.7	nil	n/a
Orange Jelly, ready to eat	Rowntree	78.0	Tr	19.6	Tr	0.6
Orange Juice	Britvic 55	49.0	0.3	11.3	Tr	n/a
	Cawston Vale	43.0	0.6	10.5	Tr	n/a
Orange Juice, unsweetened		36.0	0.5	8.8	0.1	0.1
Orange Maid, each	Lyons Maid	78.0	0.3	19.1	nil	n/a
Orange Matchmakers	Nestlé Rowntree	476	5.1	68.5	20.2	n/a
Orange Milk Chocolate	Cadbury	525	7.8	56.8	29.4	n/a

All amounts given per 100g/100ml unless otherwise stated

Product	Brand	Calories kcal	Protein (g)	Carbo-hydrate (g)	Fat (g)	Dietary Fibre (g)
Orange Mr Men, each	Lyons Maid	28.0	nil	7.0	nil	n/a
Orange Peach Apricot Juice	Del Monte	44.0	0.6	9.9	Tr	n/a
Oranges, flesh only		37.0	1.1	8.5	0.1	1.7
Orange Snack Sandwich	Cadbury	525	7.2	62.6	27.2	n/a
Orange Sorbet	Del Monte	125	0.2	32.1	Tr	n/a
Orange Special R	Robinsons	7.8	0.2	0.7	Tr	n/a
ready to drink	Robinsons	5.6	0.1	1.0	Tr	n/a
Orange Squash, low calorie	Dietade	12.0	nil	2.4	Tr	n/a
Orange Squash, undiluted	St Clements	120	0.7	31.8	0.1	n/a
Orange Whole Fruit Drink	Robinsons	47.0	0.1	10.0	Tr	n/a
Orange Yogurt	Ski	88.0	5.0	16.4	0.7	nil
Orange YoYo	McVitie's	523	4.7	63.8	27.6	1.0
Orbit Chewing Gum, sugarfree						
for Children	Wrigley	160	nil	N	nil	nil
Peppermint	Wrigley	195	nil	N	nil	nil

Spearmint	Wrigley	190	nil	N	nil	nil
Orchards Pie	McVitie's	272	3.8	38.4	12.0	1.1
Oregano, fresh		66.0	2.2	9.7	2.0	N
dried, ground		306	11.0	49.5	10.3	N
Organic Chocolate Dessert	Provamel	105	3.0	19.4	1.7	1.7
Organic Coconut & Chocolate Chip Flapjack	Doves Farm	467	5.9	52.3	26.0	4.3
Organic Crunchy Cereal	Jordans	438	10.1	57.2	18.7	7.8
Organic Hot Chocolate	Green & Black's	376	7.6	76.8	9.2	nil
Organic Lemon Cookies	Doves Farm	477	3.1	62.4	21.5	1.3
Organic Muesli	Jordans	378	10.4	54.2	13.3	10.1
Organic Oats	Mornflake	364	11.8	62.0	7.6	7.2
Organic Sliced Beets	Baxters	47.0	1.5	9.9	0.1	1.2
Organic Soya Milk, no added sugar	Provamel	36.0	36.0	0.6	2.1	1.0

All amounts given per 100g/100ml unless otherwise stated

Product	*Brand*	*Calories kcal*	*Protein (g)*	*Carbo-hydrate (g)*	*Fat (g)*	*Dietary Fibre (g)*
Organic Soya Milk with Wheat Syrup	Provamel	51.0	36.0	4.3	2.1	1.0
Organic Traditional Butter Flapjack	Doves Farm	422	5.7	55.0	19.9	3.2
Organic Vanilla Dessert	Provamel	105	3.0	19.1	1.8	1.0
Oriental Beef Stir Fry Mix, as sold	Crosse & Blackwell	350	9.0	66.0	5.3	1.1
Oriental Beef 3 Minute Noodles	Crosse & Blackwell	340	14.7	64.7	2.3	3.2
Oriental Chicken Stir Fry Mix, as sold	Crosse & Blackwell	335	6.1	70.9	2.8	0.4
Oriental Mix	Ross	43.0	2.0	9.4	0.3	1.3
Oriental Spices Seasoning Cube for Stir Fry	Knorr	409	9.5	23.7	30.7	2.7
Oriental Sweet & Sour Chicken Tonight Sauce	Batchelors	92.0	0.6	20.9	0.7	0.9

Oriental Sweet & Sour Cooking Sauce	Heinz Weight Watchers	51.0	0.8	11.7	0.1	0.8
Original Barbecue Sauce	Heinz	123	1.3	28.5	0.4	0.4
Original Beef Granules, as sold	Oxo	313	10.2	57.2	48	1.0
Original Cider	H P Bulmer	40.0	n/a	n/a	n/a	n/a
Original Energy Tablets	Lucozade Sport	361	nil	89.2	nil	n/a
Original Mallow	Jacob's	379	3.8	67.5	10.4	2.3
Original Mixed Vegetables	Birds Eye	46.0	2.9	7.5	0.5	3.1
Original Oatcakes, each	Vessen	115	2.9	15.3	4.5	1.6
Original Oatso Simple	Quaker	372	11.0	62.0	8.5	7.0
Original Pasta Sauce	Dolmio	37.0	0.9	8.4	Tr	n/a
Lite	Dolmio	24.0	0.8	5.2	Tr	n/a
with Mushrooms	Dolmio	36.0	0.9	7.9	Tr	n/a
with Spicy Peppers	Dolmio	36.0	0.9	8.2	Tr	n/a
Original Ryvita, per slice	Ryvita	27.0	0.8	5.7	0.1	1.6

All amounts given per 100g/100ml unless otherwise stated

Product	*Brand*	*Calories kcal*	*Protein (g)*	*Carbo-hydrate (g)*	*Fat (g)*	*Dietary Fibre (g)*
Original Scooples	Kavli	380	13.9	77.9	1.4	3.0
Original Vegetable Rice	Birds Eye	105	4.0	20.8	0.6	1.1
Ovaltine, powder		358	9.0	79.4	2.7	N
made up with whole milk		97.0	3.8	12.9	3.8	Tr
made up with semi-skimmed milk		79.0	3.9	13.0	1.7	Tr
Oven Chips	Ross	131	2.4	20.6	5.1	1.6
	McCain	154	1.9	26.9	4.3	n/a
Oven Crispy Cod Steaks, each	Birds Eye	240	13.0	13.0	15.0	1.3
Oven Crispy Fish Fingers	Birds Eye	218	10.4	15.8	12.6	0.4
Oven Crispy Haddock Steaks, each	Birds Eye	255	13.0	17.0	15.0	0.6
Oven Crunchies	Ross	188	2.7	24.5	8.7	1.9
Oxo Cubes: ***see individual flavours***						
Oxtail, stewed		243	30.5	nil	13.4	nil

Oxtail Cup-A-Soup, per sachet	Batchelors	76.0	1.5	13.7	1.7	1.0
Oxtail Soup, dried, as served		27.0	1.4	3.9	0.8	N
Oxtail Soup, dried, as sold		356	17.6	51.0	10.5	N
canned	Campbell's	40.0	1.4	5.3	1.5	n/a
	Heinz	41.0	1.9	6.7	0.8	0.3

All amounts given per 100g/100ml unless otherwise stated

P

Product	*Brand*	*Calories kcal*	*Protein (g)*	*Carbo-hydrate (g)*	*Fat (g)*	*Dietary Fibre (g)*
Pacific Salmon Slices	Young's	182	18.4	nil	12.0	nil
Paella, as sold	Vesta	349	10.9	69.6	2.9	3.0
Fast Cook	Ross	93.0	5.6	15.6	1.4	0.9
Paella Create-a-Stir	Findus	130	6.2	22.4	1.9	1.4
Paglia e Fieno, as sold	Dolmio	125	4.6	25.6	1.2	n/a
Pale Ale, bottled		32.0	0.3	2.0	Tr	nil
Paleskin Peanuts	Holland & Barrett	564	25.5	12.5	46.1	6.2

All amounts given per 100g/100ml unless otherwise stated

Product	*Brand*	*Calories kcal*	*Protein (g)*	*Carbo-hydrate (g)*	*Fat (g)*	*Dietary Fibre (g)*
Palm Oil		899	Tr	nil	99.9	nil
Pancake Mix	Whitworths	322	13.4	65.9	2.5	2.3
Pancake Roll		217	6.6	20.9	12.5	N
Pancakes						
savoury, made with whole milk		273	6.3	24.0	17.5	0.8
sweet, made with whole milk		301	5.9	35.0	16.2	0.8
Papaya, unripe, raw		27.0	0.9	5.5	0.1	1.5
Parmarosa Pastaria Sauce	Knorr	410	8.3	45.7	21.5	3.4
Parmesan Cheese		452	39.4	Tr	32.7	nil
	Napolina	480	44.7	Tr	33.4	n/a
Parsley & Garlic Herb Cubes	Knorr	418	8.6	34.2	27.4	1.8
Parsley Sauce Mix, as sold	Colman's	320	10.4	66.0	1.7	n/a
	Knorr	484	4.5	42.9	32.7	0.8
Parsnip & Carrot Soup	Heinz Weight Watchers	25.0	0.5	5.3	0.2	0.9

Parsnip, boiled		66.0	1.6	12.9	1.2	4.7
Partridge, roast, meat only		212	36.7	nil	7.2	nil
Passionfruit, flesh & pips only		36.0	2.6	5.8	0.4	3.3
Papaya & Passionfruit Yogurt	St Ivel Shape	55.0	5.3	7.1	0.2	0.2
Pasta Bows & Spicy Pepperoni, as sold	Findus	115	3.8	12.1	5.6	0.7
Pasta, cooked, all shapes						
egg	Buitoni	132	5.2	24.4	1.5	1.3
standard	Buitoni	129	4.8	25.9	0.7	1.2
verdi	Buitoni	127	5.0	25.2	0.7	1.3
Pasta Bolognese Dry Mix, as sold	Crosse & Blackwell	275	11.4	42.1	6.3	2.7
Pasta Choice (Crosse & Blackwell): ***see individual flavours***						
Pasta Sauce, tomato based		47.0	2.0	6.9	1.5	N
Pasta Shells with Tuna & Sweetcorn in Tomato Sauce	Heinz	79.0	5.1	10.7	1.8	0.6

All amounts given per 100g/100ml unless otherwise stated

Product	Brand	Calories kcal	Protein (g)	Carbo-hydrate (g)	Fat (g)	Dietary Fibre (g)
Pasta Tuna Provençale Dry Mix, as sold	Crosse & Blackwell	320	8.9	52.9	6.8	1.2
Pasties: *see individual flavours*						
Pastilles		253	5.2	61.9	nil	nil
Pastries: *see individual flavours*						
Pastry						
flaky, cooked		560	5.6	45.9	40.6	1.4
shortcrust, cooked		521	6.6	54.2	32.3	2.2
wholemeal, cooked		499	8.9	44.6	32.9	6.3
Pâté: *see individual flavours*						
Patent Cornflour	Brown & Polson	343	0.6	83.6	0.7	0.1
Pavlova: *see individual flavours*						
Paw-paw, raw		36.0	0.5	8.8	0.1	2.2
canned in juice		65.0	0.2	17.0	Tr	0.7
Paxo Apple & Herb Stuffing Mix	Centura	151	3.5	28.8	2.4	2.5

Paxo Chestnut & Cranberry Stuffing Mix	Centura	141	4.0	26.7	2.0	2.4
Paxo Golden Crumbs	Centura	351	11.0	72.5	1.9	5.1
Paxo Parsley, Thyme &Lemon Stuffing Mix	Centura	138	3.9	26.1	2.0	2.1
Paxo Sage & Onion Stuffing Mix	Centura	150	4.5	27.1	2.6	2.4
Paxo Traditional Chestnut Stuffing Mix	Centura	139	3.9	27.0	1.7	2.6
Pea & Ham Soup	Baxters	58.0	2.9	8.1	1.6	1.2
Peach & Banana Yogurt	St Ivel Shape	59.0	5.3	8.1	0.2	0.1
Peach & Vanilla Yogurt, per pack	Boots Shapers	61.0	n/a	n/a	0.1	n/a
Peach Chutney	Sharwood	163	0.7	39.8	0.1	2.1
Peach Dessert Mousse	St Ivel Shape	56.0	3.8	4.1	2.3	0.1
Peaches						
raw		33.0	1.0	7.6	0.1	1.5

All amounts given per 100g/100ml unless otherwise stated

Product	*Brand*	*Calories kcal*	*Protein (g)*	*Carbo-hydrate (g)*	*Fat (g)*	*Dietary Fibre (g)*
Peaches (continued)						
canned in natural juice		39.0	0.6	9.7	Tr	0.8
	Del Monte	49.0	0.5	11.2	0.1	n/a
canned in syrup		55.0	0.5	14.0	Tr	0.9
	Del Monte	77.0	0.4	18.5	0.1	n/a
Peach Fromage Frais	Ski	124	6.2	14.2	4.8	n/a
Peach Halves in Natural Juice	Libby	51.0	0.4	12.4	Tr	0.3
in Syrup	Libby	82.0	0.5	20.0	Tr	0.3
Peach Melba Ice Cream	Lyons Maid	94.0	1.7	13.2	3.8	n/a
Peach Melba Split Sundae, per pack	Boots Shapers	82.0	n/a	n/a	4.2	n/a
Peach Slices in Natural Juice	Libby	52.0	0.4	12.4	0.1	0.3
in Syrup	Libby	82.0	0.4	20.0	Tr	0.3
Peach Spring	Boots Shapers	1.0	n/a	n/a	Tr	n/a
Peach Yogurt	Ski	94.0	5.1	17.0	1.1	nil
	St Ivel	57.0	5.3	7.6	0.2	0.1

Peanut Bar, each	Boots Shapers	98.0	n/a	n/a	3.8	n/a
Peanut Butter & Chocolate Spread	Sun Pat	596	16.0	34.0	44.0	2.0
Peanut Butter, Smooth		623	22.6	13.1	53.7	5.4
	Sun Pat	615	27.8	12.0	50.5	6.5
Crunchy	Sun Pat	630	26.6	12.6	52.8	6.5
Peanut Lion Bar	Nestlé Rowntree	488	9.0	59.5	23.8	n/a
Peanut M & Ms	Mars	514	10.2	57.3	27.1	n/a
Peanut Oil		899	Tr	nil	99.9	nil
Peanuts						
plain, kernel only		564	25.6	12.5	46.1	6.2
dry roasted		589	25.5	10.3	49.8	6.4
roasted & salted		602	24.5	7.1	53.0	6.0
Peanuts & Raisins	Holland & Barrett	473	17.8	31.8	30.6	4.8
Pear & Apple Juice	Copella	39.0	n/a	10.1	nil	nil
Pear & Guava Bio Yogurt	St Ivel	56.0	5.3	7.3	0.2	0.2

All amounts given per 100g/100ml unless otherwise stated

Product	*Brand*	*Calories kcal*	*Protein (g)*	*Carbo-hydrate (g)*	*Fat (g)*	*Dietary Fibre (g)*
Pear Drops	Cravens	386	Tr	96.4	nil	nil
	Trebor Bassett	385	nil	95.4	nil	nil
Pear Halves in Syrup	Libby	77.0	0.1	19.2	Tr	0.6
in Natural Juice	Libby	54.0	0.1	13.3	Tr	0.5
Pearl Barley	Whitworths	360	7.9	83.6	1.7	7.3
Pears						
raw, average		40.0	0.3	10.0	0.1	2.2
canned in natural juice		33.0	0.3	8.5	Tr	1.4
	Del Monte	45.0	0.3	10.5	0.1	n/a
canned in syrup		50.0	0.2	13.2	Tr	1.1
	Del Monte	70.0	0.2	17.0	0.1	n/a
Peas						
boiled		79.0	6.7	10.0	1.6	4.5
dried, boiled		109	6.9	19.9	0.8	5.5
frozen, boiled		69.0	6.0	9.7	0.9	5.1
canned		80.0	5.3	13.5	0.9	5.1
Peas & Baby Carrots	Birds Eye	52.0	3.9	7.9	0.5	3.9

Pea with Ham Cup Soup	Knorr	405	9.2	49.1	19.1	1.3
Pecan and Maple Crisp	Mornflake	468	8.2	64.8	19.5	3.7
Pecan Nuts		689	9.2	5.8	70.1	4.7
Pecan Toast	Jacob's	397	11.0	72.1	7.2	5.2
Peeled Plum Tomatoes	Napolina	12.0	1.1	2.0	Tr	n/a
Peking Sizzle & Stir Sauce	Batchelors	121	0.8	9.4	8.9	1.6
Penguin Biscuits	McVitie's	448	5.3	70.0	16.5	1.1
Peperami Hot	Van den Bergh	554	19.0	2.5	52.0	1.2
Peperami Pork Salami Sausage	Van den Bergh	536	22.0	1.7	49.0	0.1
Peppercorn Mustard	Colman's	182	8.8	12.0	10.0	4.9
Peppercorn Pâté, per pack	Boots Shapers	140	n/a	n/a	8.3	n/a
Peppered Grillsteak	Ross	311	15.3	1.7	27.0	nil
Peppermint Cream	Cadbury	425	2.6	68.8	15.4	n/a
Peppermints		392	0.5	102.2	0.7	nil

All amounts given per 100g/100ml unless otherwise stated

Product	*Brand*	*Calories kcal*	*Protein (g)*	*Carbo-hydrate (g)*	*Fat (g)*	*Dietary Fibre (g)*
Pepperoni & Sausage Pizza	San Marco	226	10.9	24.8	9.9	1.3
Pepperoni Deep Crust Pizza Slices	McCain	229	10.1	26.8	9.0	n/a
Pepperoni Feast Deep Pizza	McCain	218	10.5	27.0	8.3	n/a
Pepperoni Pizza Slice	McCain	229	10.1	26.8	9.0	n/a
Pepper Pâté	Tartex	242	7.0	13.0	18.5	n/a
per tub	Vessen	97.0	2.7	4.1	7.8	0.2
Peppers						
green, raw		15.0	0.8	2.6	0.3	1.6
green, boiled		18.0	1.0	2.6	0.5	1.8
red, raw		32.0	1.0	6.4	0.4	1.6
red, boiled		34.0	1.1	7.0	0.4	1.7
yellow, raw		26.0	1.2	5.3	0.2	1.7
Pepsi	Pepsi	47.0	nil	n/a	nil	n/a
Diet Pepsi	Pepsi	0.3	n/a	n/a	nil	n/a
Pepsi Max	Pepsi	0.6	n/a	n/a	n/a	n/a

Pesto Dressing for Pasta Salads	Crosse & Blackwell	105	1.3	8.7	7.4	0.2
Petits Pois, frozen, boiled		49.0	5.0	5.5	0.9	4.5
canned		45.0	5.2	4.9	0.6	4.3
Petit Pois	Ross	51.0	4.2	10.4	1.2	4.6
Pheasant, roast, meat only		213	32.2	nil	9.3	nil
Philadelphia Full Fat Soft Cheese	Kraft	280	6.0	2.5	27.5	0.1
Philadelphia Light Medium Fat Soft Cheese	Kraft	190	8.5	3.5	16.0	0.4
with Chives	Kraft	189	9.0	3.5	15.0	0.7
with Garlic & Herbs	Kraft	181	8.7	3.5	15.0	0.7
with Ham	Kraft	186	8.8	4.4	15.0	0.4
Piccalilli	Heinz Speciality	89.0	1.2	20.5	0.3	0.5
Pickle, sweet		134	0.6	34.4	0.3	1.2
Pickled Beetroot: *see Beetroot*						
Pickled Gherkin: *see Gherkins*						

All amounts given per 100g/100ml unless otherwise stated

Product	*Brand*	*Calories kcal*	*Protein (g)*	*Carbo-hydrate (g)*	*Fat (g)*	*Dietary Fibre (g)*
Pickled Onion Crisps, per pack	Golden Wonder	131	1.4	12.3	8.5	1.1
Pickled Onions: *see Onions*						
Picnic	Cadbury	475	7.6	58.6	22.7	n/a
Pigeon, roast, meat only		230	27.8	nil	13.2	nil
Pikelets	Sunblest	194	5.8	41.0	0.7	1.6
Pilau Delicately Flavoured Rice	Batchelors	369	7.9	79.6	3.5	5.0
Pilau Rice	Sharwood	353	8.6	76.8	1.2	1.8
frozen	Uncle Ben's	148	3.4	30.5	1.4	n/a
Pilau Seasoning Cubes for Rice	Knorr	313	12.4	12.4	23.7	2.2
Pilchards, canned in tomato sauce		126	18.8	0.7	5.4	Tr
Pina Colada, per pack	Boots Shapers	33.0	n/a	n/a	nil	n/a

Pineapple						
raw		41.0	0.4	10.1	0.2	1.2
canned in natural juice		47.0	0.3	12.2	Tr	0.5
canned in syrup		64.0	0.5	16.5	Tr	0.7
Pineapple & Cream Mivi, each	Lyons Maid	85.0	1.0	13.8	2.8	n/a
Pineapple & Grapefruit Drink	Boots Shapers	2.0	n/a	n/a	Tr	n/a
Pineapple 'C'	Libby	44.0	0.1	10.9	Tr	Tr
Pineapple Chunks	Trebor Bassett	384	nil	95.1	nil	nil
Pineapple Cottage Cheese	St Ivel Shape	73.0	9.8	8.0	0.2	0.1
Pineapple Crusha	Burgess	101	Tr	24.4	nil	nil
Pineapple Fruit Juice	Del Monte	52.0	0.4	12.0	Tr	n/a
Pineapple in own Juice	Del Monte	57.0	0.4	13.0	0.1	n/a
Pineapple Juice	Britvic 55	52.0	0.2	12.1	Tr	n/a
Pineapple Juice, unsweetened		41.0	0.3	10.5	0.1	Tr

All amounts given per 100g/100ml unless otherwise stated

Product	*Brand*	*Calories kcal*	*Protein (g)*	*Carbo-hydrate (g)*	*Fat (g)*	*Dietary Fibre (g)*
Pineapple Rings						
in natural juice	Libby	50.0	n/a	n/a	Tr	n/a
in syrup	Libby	80.0	0.4	19.6	Tr	0.4
Pineapple Sorbet	Del Monte	120	0.3	30.6	Tr	n/a
Pineapple Yogurt	Ski	96.0	5.0	17.4	1.1	nil
Pine Nuts		688	14.0	4.0	68.6	1.9
Pink Grapefruit Dessert Mousse	St Ivel Shape	58.0	3.8	4.5	2.3	0.1
Pinto Beans, dried, boiled		137	8.9	23.9	0.7	N
refried		107	6.2	15.3	1.1	N
Pistachio Nuts, weighed with shells		331	9.9	4.6	30.5	3.3
Pitta Bread, white		265	9.2	57.9	1.2	2.2
Pizza: *see flavours*						
Pizza Bases (Napolina): *see individual sizes*						
Pizza Cheese Xtreme Dipz	Primula	318	12.2	29.8	16.7	n/a

Pizza Cheese Xtreme Sqeez	Primula	298	13.9	8.2	23.3	n/a
Pizza Toppings Tomato, Cheese, Onion & Herbs	Napolina	80.0	3.0	8.1	4.0	0.9
Pizza Topping, Tomato, Herbs & Spices	Napolina	67.0	1.5	9.4	2.6	0.8
PK Chewing Gum, all flavours	Wrigley	353	nil	N	nil	nil
Plaice, steamed		93.0	18.9	nil	1.9	nil
in batter, fried in oil		279	15.8	14.4	18.0	N
in crumbs, fried, fillets		228	18.0	8.6	13.7	N
Plain Chocolate		525	4.7	64.8	29.2	N
Plain Wholewheat Flapjack	Holland & Barrett	490	5.3	54.9	27.7	2.1
Ploughman's Pickle	Heinz	114	0.8	27.3	0.2	1.0
Sauces, Pickles, etc. (Heinz): ***see individual flavours***						
Plum & Blackcurrant Twinpot Yogurt	St Ivel Shape	58.0	4.5	8.8	0.1	0.2

All amounts given per 100g/100ml unless otherwise stated

Product	*Brand*	*Calories kcal*	*Protein (g)*	*Carbo-hydrate (g)*	*Fat (g)*	*Dietary Fibre (g)*
Plum Bar	Jacob's Vitalinea	370	3.6	71.9	7.5	2.3
Plum Chinese Spare Rib Sauce	Sharwood	241	0.5	59.4	0.2	0.6
Plum Sauce	Amoy	211	0.5	51.9	0.2	n/a
Straight to Wok	Amoy	246	0.2	61.0	0.2	n/a
Plums, average, raw		36.0	0.6	8.8	0.1	1.6
canned in syrup		59.0	0.3	15.5	Tr	0.8
Polo Fruits	Nestlé Rowntree	383	nil	96.0	nil	n/a
Butter-ups	Nestlé Rowntree	396	nil	93.0	2.7	n/a
Citrus Sharp	Nestlé Rowntree	393	nil	96.6	1.0	n/a
Super Ojays	Nestlé Rowntree	245	nil	96.0	1.2	nil
Polo Gummies	Nestlé Rowntree	326	7.1	75.0	Tr	n/a
Polo Mints	Nestlé Rowntree	402	nil	98.2	1.0	n/a
Sugar-Free	Nestlé Rowntree	238	nil	99.1	nil	nil
Super Mints	Nestlé Rowntree	227	nil	94.6	nil	nil

Polony		281	9.4	14.2	21.1	N
Pontefract Cakes	Trebor Bassett	278	2.2	66.6	0.3	0.7
Popcorn, candied		480	2.1	77.6	20.0	N
plain		592	6.2	48.6	42.8	N
	Holland & Barrett	592	6.2	42.8	42.8	Tr
Popcorn Prawns	Lyons Seafoods	280	9.1	18.9	19.4	n/a
Poppadums, fried in veg. oil		369	17.5	39.1	16.9	N
	Sharwood	281	20.4	45.6	1.9	10.3
Poppets Peanut	G. Payne & Co	544	16.4	37.0	37.0	n/a
Poppets Peanut & Raisin	G. Payne & Co	460	10.0	53.0	24.5	n/a
Poppets Raisins	G. Payne & Co	409	4.8	66.0	14.0	n/a
Poppets White Choc.Raisins	G. Payne & Co	286	5.9	63.6	16.6	n/a
Pork, belly rashers lean & fat, grilled		398	21.1	nil	34.8	nil
Pork, chops loin, lean only, grilled		226	32.3	nil	10.7	nil

All amounts given per 100g/100ml unless otherwise stated

Product	Brand	Calories kcal	Protein (g)	Carbo-hydrate (g)	Fat (g)	Dietary Fibre (g)
Pork, leg						
lean & fat, roast		286	26.9	nil	19.8	nil
lean only, roast		185	30.7	nil	6.9	nil
Pork, trotters & tails salted, boiled		280	19.8	nil	22.3	nil
Pork Casserole Mix, as sold	Colman's	299	5.2	67.0	0.6	n/a
Pork Pie, individual		376	9.8	24.9	27.0	0.9
Pork Sausage Casserole, as sold	Findus Red Box	80.0	2.5	7.7	4.5	1.3
Pork Sausages: *see Sausages*						
Pork Stock Cubes	Knorr	339	12.1	17.2	24.6	0.2
Porridge, made with water		49.0	1.5	9.0	1.0	0.8
made with whole milk		116	4.8	13.7	5.1	0.8
Porridge Oats	Whitworths	401	12.4	72.8	8.7	7.0

Port		157	0.1	12.0	nil	nil
Postman Pat Chew	Trebor Bassett	396	0.7	83.8	6.1	nil
Potato & Leek Soup	Baxters	40.0	1.0	6.3	1.2	0.5
Potato Crisps		546	5.6	49.3	37.6	4.9
low fat		483	6.6	63.0	21.5	6.3
Potato Croquettes, fried in oil		214	3.7	21.6	13.1	1.3
Potato, Leek & Peppers Soup	Campbell's	40.0	0.7	4.9	2.0	n/a
Potatoes, new						
boiled		75.0	1.5	17.8	0.3	1.1
boiled in skins		66.0	1.4	15.4	0.3	1.5
canned		63.0	1.5	15.1	0.1	0.8
Potatoes, old						
baked, flesh & skin		136	3.9	31.7	0.2	2.7
baked, flesh only		77.0	2.2	18.0	0.1	1.4
boiled		72.0	1.8	17.0	0.1	1.2
mashed with margarine & milk		104	1.8	15.5	4.3	1.1
roast in oil/lard		149	2.9	25.9	4.5	1.8

All amounts given per 100g/100ml unless otherwise stated

Product	*Brand*	*Calories kcal*	*Protein (g)*	*Carbo-hydrate (g)*	*Fat (g)*	*Dietary Fibre (g)*
Potato Gratin Dry Mix, as sold	Crosse & Blackwell	470	4.3	42.8	31.5	0.3
Potato Hoops		523	3.9	58.5	32.0	2.6
Potato Pancakes	Ross	239	3.2	18.8	17.4	1.3
Potato Pancakes with Onion	Ross	228	2.9	22.0	15.2	2.2
Potato Powder: *see Instant Potato Powder*						
Potato Salad	Heinz	141	1.4	14.8	8.5	0.8
Potato Waffles, frozen, cooked		200	3.2	30.3	8.2	2.3
	Ross	225	2.3	22.0	12.3	2.0
	Birds Eye	168	2.0	20.7	8.6	2.0
Potato with Broccoli, Cheese & Croutons Snack Stop	Crosse & Blackwell	96.0	2.8	9.3	5.3	n/a
Potato with Croutons & Roast Onions Snack Stop	Cross & Blackwell	109	1.8	9.0	7.3	n/a
Potted Shrimps	Young's	358	16.5	nil	32.4	nil

Pouring Syrup (Lyle's): ***see individual flavours***

Prawn & Salad Vegetables Sandwich Filler	Heinz	129	4.4	9.5	8.1	0.6
Prawn Cocktail	Lyons Seafoods	429	5.7	4.5	42.9	n/a
Prawn Cocktail Crisps, per bag	Golden Wonder	130	1.5	12.3	8.4	1.1
Prawn Cocktail Salad with Marie Rose Mayonnaise Sandwich, per pack	Boots Shapers	296	17.0	30.0	12.0	4.9
Prawn Cocktail Sandwich	Heinz Weight Watchers	145	8.9	16.6	4.8	2.5
Prawn Cocktail Sauce	Burgess	336	2.3	20.1	26.6	0.8
Prawn Cocktail Wotsits, per pack	Golden Wonder	111	1.4	11.8	6.4	0.2
Prawn Crackers	Sharwood	296	1.0	69.4	0.5	1.7
Prawn Curry as sold	Ross	117	5.0	21.5	1.4	0.4
	Findus Red Box	115	4.4	18.3	2.4	0.8

All amounts given per 100g/100ml unless otherwise stated

Product	*Brand*	*Calories kcal*	*Protein (g)*	*Carbo-hydrate (g)*	*Fat (g)*	*Dietary Fibre (g)*
Prawn Curry (continued) with rice, per pack	Birds Eye	440	13.0	78.0	8.4	3.8
Prawn Kievs	Lyons Seafoods	224	9.1	16.0	13.8	n/a
Prawn Mayonnaise Sandwich, per pack	Boots Shapers	306	15.0	30.0	14.0	5.2
Prawns, boiled		107	22.6	nil	1.8	nil
	Lyons Seafoods	61.0	13.5	nil	0.6	n/a
Prawns in Thousand Island Dressing Layered Cottage Cheese	St Ivel	146	12.8	3.6	8.8	Tr
Premier Protein Biscuit Cakes	Itona	500	15.0	50.0	26.0	n/a
Premier Protein Chocolate Biscuit Cakes	Itona	530	13.1	47.0	32.2	n/a
Premium Choice Broccoli Spears	Ross	24.0	2.9	4.1	0.7	2.6

Premium Choice Brussels Sprouts	Ross	35.0	4.1	6.6	0.5	3.2
Premium Lemonade	R Whites	26.0	Tr	6.2	Tr	n/a
Premium Scampi Tails	Lyons Seafoods	230	8.4	26.0	10.9	n/a
Preserving Sugar	Tate & Lyle	400	nil	99.9	nil	nil
Pretzel Flipz	Nestlé Rowntree	470	7.9	66.4	19.2	n/a
Primavera Pasta Express Sauce	Buitoni	70.0	1.5	6.3	4.2	n/a
Processed Cheese, plain		330	20.8	0.9	27.0	nil
Processed Peas, canned		99.0	6.9	17.5	0.7	4.8
Profiteroles	McVitie's	358	6.2	18.5	29.2	0.4
Provenzale Pasta Express Sauce	Buitoni	70.0	1.5	6.7	4.2	n/a
Prunes						
canned in juice		79.0	0.7	19.7	0.2	2.4
canned in syrup		90.0	0.6	23.0	0.2	2.8
ready to eat		141	2.5	34.0	0.4	5.7

All amounts given per 100g/100ml unless otherwise stated

Product	*Brand*	*Calories kcal*	*Protein (g)*	*Carbo-hydrate (g)*	*Fat (g)*	*Dietary Fibre (g)*
Puffed Wheat		321	14.2	67.3	1.3	5.6
Pumpkin, raw		13.0	0.7	2.2	0.2	1.0
boiled		13.0	0.6	2.1	0.3	1.1
Pumpkin Seeds	Holland & Barrett	571	29.0	47.0	n/a	n/a

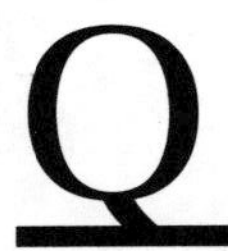

Product	Brand	Calories kcal	Protein (g)	Carbo-hydrate (g)	Fat (g)	Dietary Fibre (g)
Quaker Oat Bran Crispies	Quaker	370	12.2	68.8	4.6	9.0
Quaker Oat Crunch	Quaker	445	8.0	66.5	16.0	5.0
Quaker Oats	Quaker	368	11.0	62.0	8.0	7.0
Quaker Puffed Wheat	Quaker	328	15.3	62.4	1.3	5.6
Quality Street	Nestlé Rowntree	461	3.6	66.7	20.0	0.8
Quarter Pounder, each	McDonald's	423	25.7	37.1	19.0	3.7
with cheese, each	McDonald's	516	31.2	37.5	26.7	3.7

All amounts given per 100g/100ml unless otherwise stated

Product	Brand	Calories kcal	Protein (g)	Carbo-hydrate (g)	Fat (g)	Dietary Fibre (g)
Quiche						
cheese & egg		314	12.5	17.3	22.2	0.6
cheese & egg, wholemeal		308	13.2	14.5	22.4	1.9
Quorn, myco-protein		86.0	11.8	2.0	3.5	4.8
Quosh Fruit Drinks: ***see individual flavours***						

R

Product	*Brand*	*Calories kcal*	*Protein (g)*	*Carbo-hydrate (g)*	*Fat (g)*	*Dietary Fibre (g)*
Rabbit, stewed, meat only		179	27.3	nil	7.7	nil
Raddiccio, raw		14.0	1.4	1.7	0.2	1.8
Radish, red, raw		12.0	0.7	1.9	0.2	0.9
white/mooli, raw		15.0	0.8	2.9	0.1	N
Ragu Pasta Sauces: *see individual flavours*						
Rainbow Trout	Young's	89.0	13.8	nil	3.8	nil
Raisin & Almond Original Crunchy	Jordans	402	8.7	65.3	11.8	6.4

All amounts given per 100g/100ml unless otherwise stated

Product	*Brand*	*Calories kcal*	*Protein (g)*	*Carbo-hydrate (g)*	*Fat (g)*	*Dietary Fibre (g)*
Raisin & Biscuit Yorkie	Nestlé Rowntree	481	5.8	60.9	23.8	n/a
Raisin & Hazelnut Frusli Bar, each	Jordans	142	2.1	20.4	5.8	1.3
Raisin & Lemon Pancakes	Sunblest	274	5.8	52.6	4.5	1.4
Raisin Country Crisp	Jordans	442	7.3	65.7	16.7	5.8
Raisins		272	2.1	69.3	0.4	2.0
Raisins & Peanuts		435	15.3	37.5	26.0	4.4
Raisin Toast	Jacob's	368	13.1	70.1	3.9	4.4
Raisin Wheats	Kellogg's	320	9.0	69.0	1.5	9.0
Rambutans & Pineapple in Syrup	Libby	74.0	n/a	n/a	Tr	n/a
Ranch Dressing	Kraft	420	1.7	7.6	42.0	0.1
Ranch Dressing with Blue Cheese	Kraft	395	1.6	8.2	39.5	0.1
Rapeseed Oil		899	Tr	nil	99.9	nil

Raspberries, raw		7.0	0.9	0.8	0.1	2.5
stewed with sugar		48.0	0.9	11.5	0.1	1.2
stewed without sugar		7.0	0.9	0.7	0.1	1.3
canned in syrup		31.0	0.5	7.6	Tr	0.8
Raspberry Ripple Slices	Mr Kipling	375	2.4	52.8	15.3	n/a
Raspberry & Cream Mivi, each	Lyons Maid	84.0	1.2	13.5	2.8	n/a
Raspberry & Redcurrant Creme Brulee	McVitie's	251	1.3	23.5	17.0	0.2
Raspberr y & Vanilla Swiss Roll	Lyons Cakes	336	4.6	58.4	7.6	n/a
Raspberry Cheesecake	Young's	299	4.7	31.9	17.2	0.6
Raspberry Country Crisp	Jordans	401	7.2	58.5	15.4	5.8
Raspberry Crisp	Mornflake	439	6.8	69.6	14.8	4.0
Raspberry Crusha	Burgess	103	Tr	24.7	nil	nil
Raspberry Flavour Jelly Crystals	Dietade	8.0	1.6	0.2	nil	nil

All amounts given per 100g/100ml unless otherwise stated

Product	Brand	Calories kcal	Protein (g)	Carbo-hydrate (g)	Fat (g)	Dietary Fibre (g)
Raspberry Fruit Spread	Heinz Weight Watchers	111	0.4	27.1	0.1	0.9
Raspberry Jam, sucrose free	Dietade	259	0.5	63.9	0.1	n/a
Raspberry Jelly, ready to eat	Rowntree	81.0	0.1	20.2	Tr	0.8
Raspberry Organic Jam	Baxters	252	Tr	63.0	Tr	1.2
Raspberry Pavlova	McVitie's	297	2.5	45.0	11.9	Tr
Raspberry Preserve	Baxters	210	Tr	53.0	Tr	1.2
Raspberry Ripple Ice Cream	Fiesta	192	3.2	24.3	9.8	n/a
	Lyons Maid	114	1.6	19.0	3.5	n/a
Raspberry Ripple Mousse, each	Fiesta	90.0	2.0	11.4	4.0	n/a
Raspberry Swirl Iced Dessert	Heinz Weight Watchers	124	1.7	23.4	2.5	0.3
Raspberry Swiss Roll	Lyons Cakes	305	5.0	64.6	1.5	n/a
Raspberry Torte	McVitie's	271	3.5	24.5	17.8	0.4

Raspberry Trifle	St Ivel	173	2.5	21.1	8.7	0.4
luxury	St Ivel	166	2.1	21.6	7.9	0.3
	Heinz Weight Watchers	110	3.2	18.4	1.8	0.4
per pack	Boots Shapers	96.0	n/a	n/a	3.6	n/a
Raspberry Yogurt	Ski	94.0	5.1	17.0	1.1	nil
Ratatouille Dry Mix, as sold	Crosse & Blackwell	330	11.3	48.8	8.8	2.0
Ravioli Bianche, as sold	Dolmio	200	9.6	29.7	4.7	n/a
Ravioli in Tomato Sauce	Heinz	73.0	2.6	13.0	1.1	0.6
Raw Cane Demerara Sugar	Tate & Lyle	400	Tr	99.2	nil	Tr
Ready Brek	Weetabix	359	12.0	59.9	8.4	8.4
Ready Cook Casserole	Itona	45.0	1.7	7.7	0.8	n/a
Ready Salted Crisps, per pack	Golden Wonder	135	1.4	12.5	8.8	1.1
Ready to Eat Prunes	Holland & Barrett	134	2.0	33.5	Tr	13.4

All amounts given per 100g/100ml unless otherwise stated

Product	*Brand*	*Calories kcal*	*Protein (g)*	*Carbo-hydrate (g)*	*Fat (g)*	*Dietary Fibre (g)*
Real Chocloate Chip Cookies	Heinz Weight Watchers	427	5.3	66.1	15.7	1.6
Real Chocolate Mousse	Chambourcy	189	4.8	25.8	7.4	0.3
Real Mayonnaise	Burgess	717	1.4	3.0	77.5	0.4
	Hellmanns	721	1.0	1.5	79.0	nil
Real Oyster Chinese Pouring Sauce	Sharwood	75.0	1.3	17.0	0.2	0.3
Red Box (Findus): ***see individual flavours***						
Red Cherry Bio Yogurt	St Ivel	57.0	5.3	7.6	0.1	0.1
Redcurrant Jelly	Baxters	260	nil	65.0	nil	nil
	Burgess	129	0.6	31.0	nil	nil
	Colman's	368	0.7	90.0	Tr	n/a
Red Kidney Beans, boiled		103	8.4	17.4	0.5	9.0
canned		100	6.9	17.8	0.6	8.5
	Batchelors	91.0	8.1	13.5	0.5	6.4
	Holland & Barrett	262	22.1	40.2	1.4	15.7

Red Lentils: ***see Lentils***						
Red Peppers: ***see Peppers***						
Reduced Fat Spreads: ***see individual brands/flavours***						
Reduced Salt Clover	Dairy Crest	388	7.1	n/a	39.9	n/a
Red Wine		68.0	0.2	0.3	nil	nil
Red Wine & Herbs	Ragu	62.0	2.1	8.8	2.0	1.1
Red Wine Cook-In-Sauce	Homepride	48.0	0.5	10.1	0.6	n/a
Refreshers	Trebor Bassett	375	0.1	90.2	0.3	nil
Revels	Mars	495	6.2	65.6	23.1	n/a
Rhubarb, stewed with sugar		48.0	0.9	11.5	0.1	1.2
stewed without sugar		7.0	0.9	0.7	0.1	1.3
canned in syrup		31.0	0.5	7.6	Tr	0.8
Rhubarb & Custard Twinpot Yogurt	St Ivel Shape	54.0	4.6	8.0	0.1	0.1
Rhubarb & Custard Yogurt	St Ivel Shape	54.0	4.6	7.8	0.1	0.1
Rhubarb & Ginger Preserve	Baxters	210	Tr	53.0	Tr	0.6

All amounts given per 100g/100ml unless otherwise stated

Product	Brand	Calories kcal	Protein (g)	Carbo-hydrate (g)	Fat (g)	Dietary Fibre (g)
Ribena Spark	SmithKline Beecham	54.0	Tr	13.3	nil	n/a
low calorie		2.0	Tr	0.1	nil	n/a
Ribena, undiluted		228	0.1	60.8	nil	nil
Rice, boiled						
brown		141	2.6	32.1	1.1	0.8
white		138	2.6	30.9	1.3	0.1
Rice Dessert	St Ivel Shape	85.0	3.5	15.4	1.0	0.1
Rice Drink	Provamel	49.0	0.1	10.0	1.0	nil
Rice Krispies		369	6.1	89.7	0.9	0.7
	Kellogg's	370	6.0	85.0	1.0	1.5
Rice Pops	Doves Farm	362	6.6	80.6	1.5	1.7
Rice Pudding, canned		89.0	3.4	14.0	2.5	0.2
	Creamola	380	6.4	85.0	1.0	2.4
low fat, no added sugar	Heinz Weight Watchers	73.0	3.7	11.4	1.5	nil

Rich & Spicy Baste 'n' Grill Sauce	Lea & Perrins	176	1.5	43.7	0.8	n/a
Rich Chocolate Roll	Cadbury	396	4.9	52.3	16.3	n/a
Rich Fruit Cake: *see Fruit Cake*						
Rich Mediterranean Pour over Sauce	Baxters	53.0	1.2	7.9	1.9	1.4
Rich Muesli	Holland & Barrett	381	11.0	60.5	12.2	7.7
Rich Soy Chinese Pouring Sauce	Sharwood	48.0	4.6	7.5	Tr	0.3
Rich Tea Biscuits	McVitie's	470	6.7	74.2	15.7	2.3
Rich Tea Fingers	McVitie's	466	6.8	75.7	14.5	2.3
Ricicles		381	4.3	95.7	0.5	0.4
	Kellogg's	380	4.0	89.0	0.7	1.0
Ricotta and Spinach filled pasta, as sold	Findus	115	3.4	14.5	4.7	0.5

All amounts given per 100g/100ml unless otherwise stated

Product	*Brand*	*Calories kcal*	*Protein (g)*	*Carbo-hydrate (g)*	*Fat (g)*	*Dietary Fibre (g)*
Risotto Create-a-Stir	Findus	130	6.2	22.4	1.9	1.4
Risotto, plain		224	3.0	34.4	9.3	0.4
Risotto Rice	Whitworths	324	7.0	77.8	0.6	0.2
Ritz Cheese Crackers	Jacob's	470	11.0	58.0	22.0	3.0
Ritz Cheese Sandwich	Jacob's	509	8.9	52.7	29.3	1.7
Ritz Original Crackers	Jacob's	503	7.0	57.0	28.0	2.0
Roast Beef Dinner, each	Birds Eye	370	29.0	39.0	11.0	4.6
Roast Chicken Crisps, per pack	Golden Wonder	130	1.6	12.2	8.4	1.1
Roast Chicken Dinner, each	Birds Eye	385	34.0	35.0	12.0	5.1
Roast Chicken Salad with Lemon & Tarragon Mayonnaise Sandwiches, per pack	Boots Shapers	326	21.0	38.0	10.0	4.2

Roast Chicken, Tomato & Pesto with Mixed Leaf and Mayonnaise Sandwich, per pack	Boots Shapers	344	23.0	36.0	12.0	5.7
Roast Chicken with Creamy Black Pepper Mayonnaise Sandwiches, per pack	Boots Shapers	282	25.0	24.0	9.5	4.6
Roasted Red Pepper Dressing for Pasta Salads	Crosse & Blackwell	80.0	1.0	13.4	2.1	0.2
Roasted Vegetable Salsa Layered Cottage Cheese	St Ivel	80.0	9.5	5.0	2.3	0.4
Roasted Vegetables, Soft Cheese &Pesto with Mixed Leaf Sandwiches, per pack	Boots Shapers	280	12.0	38.0	8.9	3.9
Roast Lamb Dinner, each	Birds Eye	350	23.0	40.0	11.0	4.6
Roast Lamb in Gravy, per pack	Birds Eye	160	19.0	9.1	5.2	0.2

All amounts given per 100g/100ml unless otherwise stated

Product	Brand	Calories kcal	Protein (g)	Carbo-hydrate (g)	Fat (g)	Dietary Fibre (g)
Roast Nut Tracker	Mars	541	9.2	57.5	30.5	n/a
Roast Pork in Gravy, per pack	Birds Eye	145	22.0	7.5	2.5	0.2
Roast Pork Dinner, each	Birds Eye	340	27.0	39.0	8.2	5.0
Roast Turkey Dinner, each	Birds Eye	330	24.0	34.0	11.0	5.0
Roe						
cod, hard, fried		202	20.9	3.0	11.9	0.1
herring, soft, fried		244	21.1	4.7	15.8	N
Rogan Josh Classic Curry Sauce	Homepride	65.0	2.5	12.3	0.8	n/a
Rogan Josh Medium Curry Sauce	Sharwood	90.0	2.8	7.3	5.6	2.6
Rogan Josh Medium Curry Sauce mix, as sold	Sharwood	197	10.1	16.7	10.0	21.5
Rolls: ***see Bread Rolls***						
Rolo	Nestlé Rowntree	473	4.3	67.1	20.8	n/a

Rolo Dessert	Chambourcy	240	3.1	31.0	11.5	0.2
Romana Pasta Choice Mix, as sold	Crosse & Blackwell	360	12.3	59.2	7.9	3.3
Rosehip Syrup, undiluted		232	Tr	61.9	nil	nil
Roses	Cadbury	485	4.8	60.9	24.8	n/a
Rosé Wine		71.0	0.1	2.5	nil	nil
Rowntree Jelly, Tablet	Nestle					
Orange, Lemon, Lime, Blackcurrant		296	6.0	67.5	nil	nil
Strawberry, Raspberry		297	6.0	67.7	nil	nil
Pineapple, Peach		295	6.0	67.1	nil	nil
Black Cherry		289	6.0	66.0	nil	nil
Tangerine		294	6.0	67.2	nil	nil
Fruits of the Forest		300	5.9	67.6	0.5	nil
Royal Game Soup	Baxters	36.0	2.4	5.5	0.5	0.4
Royal Icing	Tate & Lyle	390	1.4	97.5	nil	nil
Royal Lemon Pie Filling Mix	Green's	390	0.5	94.5	1.4	n/a

All amounts given per 100g/100ml unless otherwise stated

Product	Brand	Calories kcal	Protein (g)	Carbo-hydrate (g)	Fat (g)	Dietary Fibre (g)
Ruby's Cranberry & Blueberry Soda	Britvic	38.0	Tr	9.0	nil	n/a
Ruby's Cranberry & Orange Soda	Britvic	40.0	Tr	9.0	Tr	n/a
Ruby's Cranberry & Raspberry Soda	Britvic	38.0	Tr	9.0	Tr	n/a
Rum: *see Spirits*						
Rum & Raisin Napoli	Lyons Maid	104	1.8	12.4	5.1	n/a
Rum Hot Chocolate, per pack	Boots Shapers	36.0	n/a	n/a	0.9	n/a
Rump Steak: *see Beef*						
Rum Sauce Mix	Bird's	415	6.1	76.5	9.5	nil
Runner Beans, boiled		18.0	1.2	2.3	0.5	3.1
Rye Bread: *see Bread*						

Rye Crispbread		321	9.4	70.6	2.1	11.7
per slice	Boots Shapers	15.0	n/a	n/a	0.1	n/a
Rye Flour, whole		335	8.2	75.9	20.	11.7
Ryvita: *see individual flavours*						

S

Product	Brand	Calories kcal	Protein (g)	Carbo-hydrate (g)	Fat (g)	Dietary Fibre (g)
Safflower Oil		899	Tr	nil	99.9	nil
Saffron Seasoning Cube for Rice	Knorr	296	13.7	15.7	19.8	3.0
Sage & Onion Stuffing		231	5.2	20.4	14.8	1.7
	Whitworths	398	5.7	73.6	9.0	1.9
Sago Pudding	Whitworths	355	0.2	94.0	0.2	nil
Saithe: *see Coley*						

All amounts given per 100g/100ml unless otherwise stated

Product	Brand	Calories kcal	Protein (g)	Carbo-hydrate (g)	Fat (g)	Dietary Fibre (g)
Salad Cream		348	1.5	16.7	31.0	N
	Heinz	327	1.4	19.8	26.8	nil
reduced calorie		194	1.0	9.4	17.2	N
light	Heinz	234	1.4	12.5	19.8	nil
Salad Mayonnaise	Burgess	579	2.4	8.1	59.2	nil
Salami		491	19.3	1.9	45.2	0.1
Salmon						
steamed, flesh only		197	20.1	nil	13.0	nil
canned		155	203.	nil	8.2	nil
smoked		142	25.4	nil	4.5	nil
Salmon Mornay with Broccoli	Heinz Weight Watchers	91.0	9.0	9.1	2.1	0.7
Salmon Spread	Shippams	221	14.5	2.5	17.1	n/a
Salsa Dippits	Primula	101	3.7	20.7	0.4	n/a
Salsify, raw		27.0	1.3	10.2	0.3	3.2
boiled		23.0	1.1	8.6	0.4	3.5

Salt & Vinegar crisps, per pack	Golden Wonder	130	1.4	12.1	8.5	1.1
Salt & Vinegar Golden Lights per pack	Golden Wonder	94.0	1.0	13.8	3.8	0.8
Salt & Vinegar Wheat Crunchies, per pack	Golden Wonder	170	3.7	19.1	8.7	0.9
Salted Cashew Nuts: *see Cashew Nuts*						
Samosas, meat		593	5.1	17.9	56.1	1.2
vegetable		472	3.1	22.3	41.8	1.8
Sandwich Biscuits		513	5.0	69.2	25.9	N
Sandwich Cake Mixes: *see individual flavours*						
Sandwich Cakes: *see individual flavours*						
Sandwich Fillers (Shippams): *see individual flavours*						
Sandwich Spread	Heinz	221	1.3	25.3	12.7	0.8
Santa Bakewells	Mr Kipling	425	3.9	62.7	17.6	n/a
Santa Snow Cakes	Lyons Cakes	449	5.6	55.2	22.3	n/a

All amounts given per 100g/100ml unless otherwise stated

Product	Brand	Calories kcal	Protein (g)	Carbo-hydrate (g)	Fat (g)	Dietary Fibre (g)
Sardine & Tomato Spread	Shippams	156	16.6	2.1	9.0	n/a
Sardines						
canned in tomato sauce		177	17.8	0.5	11.6	Tr
canned in oil, drained		217	23.7	nil	13.6	nil
Satay Sauce	Amoy	198	10.2	11.6	12.3	n/a
Satsumas, flesh only		36.0	0.9	8.5	0.1	1.3
Sauce à L'Orange Dry Mix, as sold	Crosse & Blackwell	365	1.4	76.0	5.3	0.2
Sauce Tartare: ***see Tartare Sauce***						
Sauerkraut		9.0	1.1	1.1	Tr	2.2
Sausage & Tomato Classic QuickCook Mix, as sold	Crosse & Blackwell	375	11.7	61.1	8.4	2.4
Sausage & Tomato Pasta Mix	Colman's	308	7.9	63.0	1.3	n/a
Sausage & Tomato Pot Noodle	Golden Wonder	429	11.5	62.1	15.1	3.3

Sausage Hotpot	Heinz Baked Bean Cuisine	99.0	5.2	13.3	2.7	2.5
Sausage in Onion Gravy & Mash, per pack	Birds Eye	440	17.0	40.0	24.0	3.2
Sausage, Onion and Mash Dry Mix, as sold	Crosse & Blackwell	355	9.6	58.6	8.6	1.2
Sausage Rolls						
flaky pastry		477	7.1	32.3	36.4	1.2
short pastry		459	8.0	37.5	31.9	1.4
	Ross	289	11.1	19.4	19.3	0.8
Sausages, beef						
fried		269	12.9	14.9	18.0	0.7
grilled		265	13.0	15.2	17.3	0.7
Sausages, pork						
fried		317	13.8	11.0	24.5	0.7
grilled		318	13.3	11.5	24.6	0.7
low fat, fried		211	14.9	9.1	13.0	1.4
low fat, grilled		229	16.2	10.8	1.38	1.5

All amounts given per 100g/100ml unless otherwise stated

Product	Brand	Calories kcal	Protein (g)	Carbo-hydrate (g)	Fat (g)	Dietary Fibre (g)
Saveloy		262	9.9	10.1	20.5	N
Savoury Mince	Tyne Brand	86.0	9.8	13.4	7.3	0.6
Savoury Mince Beanfeast, per packet, as served	Batchelors	316	24.7	39.5	6.6	12.7
Savoury Rice, cooked		142	2.9	26.3	3.5	1.4
Savoury Spread	Primula	261	17.0	1.0	21.0	n/a
Savoury White Sauce Mix	Knorr	357	4.9	61.6	10.2	0.2
Scampi & Lemon Nik Naks, per pack	Golden Wonder	187	2.1	19.2	11.4	0.4
Scampi in Breadcrumbs, frozen, fried		316	12.2	28.9	17.6	N
Scones, fruit		316	7.3	52.9	9.8	N
plain		362	7.2	53.8	14.6	1.9
wholemeal		326	8.7	43.1	14.4	5.2
Scotch Broth	Baxters	47.0	1.9	7.1	1.2	0.9
	Campbell's	38.0	0.9	4.5	1.8	n/a

Scotch Eggs		251	12.0	13.1	17.1	N
Scotch Orange Marmalade	Baxters	210	Tr	53.0	Tr	Tr
Scotch Pancakes		292	5.8	43.6	11.7	1.4
	Sunblest	277	6.7	50.0	5.6	1.4
Scotch Vegetable Soup	Baxters	43.0	1.9	7.4	0.6	1.3
Scotch Whisky: *see Spirits*						
Scottish Lentil Soup	Crosse & Blackwell	44.0	2.6	6.2	1.0	1.0
Scottish Plain White Bread	Sunblest	232	9.3	45.7	1.3	2.2
Scottish Salmon Side	Young's	182	18.4	nil	12.0	nil
Scottish Salmon Slices	Young's	182	18.4	nil	12.0	nil
Scottish Vegetable Soup	Campbell's	39.0	0.6	4.5	2.0	n/a
Scottish Vegetable Soup with Lentils & Beef	Heinz	52.0	3.4	8.2	0.7	1.2
Scott's Old Fashioned Porage Oats	Quaker	368	11.0	62.0	8.0	7.0

All amounts given per 100g/100ml unless otherwise stated

Product	*Brand*	*Calories kcal*	*Protein (g)*	*Carbo-hydrate (g)*	*Fat (g)*	*Dietary Fibre (g)*
Scott's Piper Oatmeal	Quaker	368	11.0	62.0	8.0	7.0
Scotts Porage Oats	Quaker	368	11.0	62.0	8.0	7.0
Scrambled Eggs: ***see Eggs***						
Seafood Cocktail	Lyons Seafoods	72.0	14.0	2.0	1.8	n/a
Seafood Crumble	Ross	197	8.7	11.3	13.2	0.5
Seafood Lasagne	Ross	117	7.2	10.7	5.3	1.0
Seafood Sauce	Baxters	533	1.5	9.9	54.2	0.7
	Colman's	335	0.9	20.0	28.0	n/a
Seafood Selection	Lyons Seafoods	81.0	14.9	1.3	2.3	n/a
	Young's	66.0	11.5	nil	2.2	nil
Seafood Sticks	Young's	97.0	10.7	14.1	0.1	nil
Seedless Raisins	Holland & Barrett	246	1.1	64.4	Tr	6.8
	Whitworths	289	2.1	69.3	0.4	2.0
Semi-skimmed Milk: ***see Milk***						

Semolina Pudding	Whitworths	350	10.7	77.5	1.8	2.1
Semolina Whisk & Serve	Bird's	440	5.1	73.3	13.0	1.1
Sesame Oil		881	0.2	nil	99.7	nil
Sesame Ryvita, per slice	Ryvita	31.0	0.9	5.3	0.6	1.4
7 Up	Pepsi	46.0	nil	n/a	nil	n/a
Diet	Pepsi	1.1	nil	n/a	nil	n/a
Seville Orange Fruit Spread	Heinz Weight Watchers	111	0.2	27.5	nil	0.3
Shandy	Barr	30.0	n/a	7.4	Tr	Tr
Shandy Bass	Britvic	22.0	Tr	4.7	nil	n/a
Shapers (Boots): ***see individual flavours***						
Shepherd's Pie	Heinz Baked Bean Cuisine	88.0	4.1	11.6	2.8	1.5
	Ross	128	4.6	14.7	5.9	0.6
per pack	Birds Eye	101	4.1	11.0	4.5	0.8
Shepherd's Pie Filling	Tyne Brand	105	7.8	5.5	5.8	n/a

All amounts given per 100g/100ml unless otherwise stated

Product	*Brand*	*Calories kcal*	*Protein (g)*	*Carbo-hydrate (g)*	*Fat (g)*	*Dietary Fibre (g)*
Shepherd's Pie Classic Creations Mix, as sold	Crosse & Blackwell	300	12.1	48.0	6.2	1.6
Sherbert Lemons	Cravens	423	Tr	89.0	7.4	nil
	Trebor Bassett	382	nil	93.9	nil	nil
Sherbet Fountain	Trebor Bassett	352	0.6	84.0	0.1	0.2
Sherbet Fruits	Cravens	423	Tr	89.0	7.4	nil
Sherry						
dry		116	0.2	1.4	nil	nil
medium		118	0.1	3.6	nil	nil
sweet		136	0.3	6.9	nil	nil
Sherry Gateau	McVitie's	329	2.8	28.8	22.6	0.1
Shortbread		498	5.9	63.9	26.1	1.9
Shortbread Biscuit	Holland & Barrett	518	4.5	64.3	27.0	Tr
Shortcake	Jacob's	488	6.7	65.4	22.1	2.0

Shortcake Snack	Cadbury	525	6.9	64.6	26.6	n/a
Shortcrust Pastry Mix	Whitworths	467	7.4	60.8	23.2	2.3
Shortcrust Pastry: *see Pastry*						
Short Grain Rice	Whitworths	361	6.5	86.8	1.0	2.4
Shredded Cabbage	Ross	19.0	1.1	5.5	0.2	2.3
Shredded Wheat		325	10.6	68.3	3.0	9.8
	Nestlé	347	11.0	70.8	2.2	9.5
Shreddies	Nestlé	353	9.8	74.2	1.9	8.3
Shrimps, frozen, without shells		73.0	16.5	nil	0.8	nil
canned, drained		94.0	20.8	nil	1.2	nil
Sicilian Pork Regional Recipes	Ragu	35.0	1.0	6.0	0.8	0.7
Silverside, Sirloin: *see Beef*						
Singapore Noodles Snackpot, as sold	Findus Lean Cuisine	90.0	2.7	15.3	1.8	1.1
Singles Cheese Slices	Kraft	290	15.5	6.2	22.5	nil

All amounts given per 100g/100ml unless otherwise stated

Product	*Brand*	*Calories kcal*	*Protein (g)*	*Carbo-hydrate (g)*	*Fat (g)*	*Dietary Fibre (g)*
Singles Light Cheese Slices	Kraft	205	20.0	6.0	11.0	nil
Skate, fried in butter		199	17.9	4.9	12.1	0.2
Skimmed Milk: *see Milk*						
Skittles	Mars	406	0.3	91.5	4.3	n/a
Skittles Fun Up	Mars	85.0	0.2	21.0	nil	n/a
Sliced Green Beans	Ross	31.0	1.8	7.6	0.2	2.2
Sliced Mushrooms, dried	Whitworths	223	16.5	40.0	1.0	22.9
Sliced Onions, dried	Whitworths	258	11.9	68.9	Tr	17.2
Small Processed Peas	Batchelors	87.0	5.4	15.5	0.4	4.8
Smarties	Nestlé Rowntree	459	5.4	71.1	17.0	n/a
Giant	Nestlé Rowntree	477	5.3	69.0	20.0	n/a
Mini	Nestlé Rowntree	455	4.2	71.5	16.9	nil
Smarties Dessert Split Pot	Chambourcy	250	4.0	35.6	9.8	n/a
Smatana	Raines	130	4.7	5.6	10.0	n/a

Smoked Haddock Cutlets	Ross	77.0	17.8	nil	0.6	nil
Smoked Haddock Fillets with Butter	Birds Eye	85.0	16.0	nil	2.3	nil
Smoked Salmon Spread	Shippams	237	13.4	5.6	17.9	n/a
Smoked Turkey, Ham & Coleslaw with lettuce Sandwiches, per pack	Boots Shapers	337	22.0	33.0	13.0	5.3
Smokey Barbecue Sauce	Heinz	89.0	1.2	20.5	0.2	0.7
Smokey Tomato Barbecue Sauce	HP	143	0.8	33.1	0.2	n/a
Smoky Bacon Crisps, per pack	Golden Wonder	131	1.5	12.3	8.4	1.1
Smooth Hot Chocolate	Boots Shapers	37.0	n/a	n/a	0.9	n/a
Smooth Peanut Butter	Sunpat	620	25.8	14.5	50.9	6.5
Snack Breakpack	Cadbury	525	7.0	64.2	26.8	n/a
Snackpack	Primula	282	14.1	18.3	14.7	n/a

All amounts given per 100g/100ml unless otherwise stated

Product	*Brand*	*Calories kcal*	*Protein (g)*	*Carbo-hydrate (g)*	*Fat (g)*	*Dietary Fibre (g)*
Snack Wafer	Cadbury	555	4.3	57.3	33.7	n/a
Snickers	Mars	510	10.2	55.3	27.6	n/a
Snickers Ice Cream Bar	Mars	381	7.8	33.3	24.1	n/a
Snowballs	Tunnock's	388	3.9	47.0	21.8	n/a
Soft Brown Rolls	Heinz Weight Watchers	216	10.7	39.3	1.8	4.1
Soft Cheese & Roasted Peppers Sandwich, low fat	Heinz Weight Watchers	181	9.7	27.0	3.9	1.5
Soft Fruit Centres	Cravens	386	Tr	96.4	nil	nil
Softfruits	Trebor Bassett	366	0.1	88.1	1.2	nil
Softmints	Trebor Bassett	374	0.1	88.2	2.3	nil
Soft White Rolls	Heinz Weight Watchers	221	10.4	41.6	1.5	3.3
Sole: *see Lemon Sole*						
Solstis	Lucozade	62.0	nil	15.0	nil	n/a

Somerset Pork Sauce, as sold	Colman's	59	0.4	7.2	3.2	0.7
Soup: *see individual flavours*						
Soup & Broth Mix	Whitworths	332	14.1	70.2	1.4	8.6
Sour Cream & Chives Crinkle Crisps	Boots Shapers	482	n/a	n/a	24.0	n/a
Sour Cream & Chive Dip	Primula	345	5.0	1.8	35.3	n/a
Sour Cream & Chives Potato Bake Mix, as sold	Colman's	405	12.1	44.5	19.7	5.2
Sour Cream and Chives Savoury Snack	Jordans	417	7.3	69.9	12.0	2.7
Sour Cream & Onion Golden Lights, per pack	Golden Wonder	94.0	1.1	13.9	3.7	0.8
Southern Fried Chicken	Birds Eye	278	14.6	13.4	18.4	0.9
Southern Fried Chicken Coat and Cook	Homepride	419	10.1	42.8	22.4	n/a
Southern Fries Savoury Herb Ranch Fries	McCain	164	2.1	25.3	6.0	n/a

All amounts given per 100g/100ml unless otherwise stated

Product	*Brand*	*Calories kcal*	*Protein (g)*	*Carbo-hydrate (g)*	*Fat (g)*	*Dietary Fibre (g)*
Southern Fries Savoury Herb Slice	McCain	158	2.1	22.4	6.7	n/a
Southern Style Chicken Crispy Pancakes	Findus	100	5.6	23.9	4.8	1.1
Southern Style Skins	McCain	147	2.2	17.8	7.4	n/a
Soya Bean Curd: ***see Tofu***						
Soya Beans, boiled		141	14.0	5.1	7.3	6.1
Soya Chunks Flavoured	Holland & Barrett	345	50.0	35.0	1.0	4.0
Unflavoured	Holland & Barrett	345	50.0	35.0	1.0	4.0
Soya Curd: ***see Tofu***						
Soya Dream	Provamel	178	3.0	1.7	17.7	1.1
Soya Milk	Provamel					
Banana flavour	Provamel	75.0	36.0	10.5	2.1	1.2

Chocolate flavour	Provamel	71.0	36.0	9.5	2.1	1.5
Strawberry flavour	Provamel	64.0	36.0	7.7	2.1	1.2
Soya Flour						
full fat		447	36.8	23.5	23.5	11.2
low fat		352	45.3	28.2	7.2	13.5
Soya Milk, plain		32.0	2.9	0.8	1.9	nil
flavoured		40.0	2.8	3.6	1.7	nil
Soya Mince Flavoured	Holland & Barrett	345	50.0	35.0	1.0	4.0
Unflavoured	Holland & Barrett	345	50.0	35.0	1.0	4.0
Soya Oil		899	Tr	nil	99.9	nil
Soya Yogurt: *see Yogurt*						
Soy Sauce, dark, thick		64.0	8.7	8.3	nil	nil
Spaghetti, cooked						
white		104	3.6	22.2	0.7	1.2
wholemeal		113	4.7	23.2	0.9	3.5

All amounts given per 100g/100ml unless otherwise stated

Product	*Brand*	*Calories kcal*	*Protein (g)*	*Carbo-hydrate (g)*	*Fat (g)*	*Dietary Fibre (g)*
Spaghetti Bolognese	Heinz	86.0	3.4	12.8	2.3	0.7
	Birds Eye	112	4.8	13.4	4.4	0.9
Spaghetti Bolognese Sauce Mix, as sold	Colman's	313	9.5	64.0	1.1	n/a
Spaghetti Hoops	Heinz	56.0	1.9	11.7	0.2	0.6
Spaghetti Hoops 'n' Hotdogs in a Smoky Bacon Sauce	Heinz	76.0	2.8	11.0	2.4	0.4
Spaghetti in Tomato Sauce	Heinz	61.0	1.7	13.0	0.2	0.5
	Crosse & Blackwell	88.0	3.3	15.0	1.7	n/a
no added sugar	Heinz Weight Watchers	50.0	1.8	10.1	0.2	0.6
Spaghetti Napoli	Findus Red Box	75.0	2.8	13.3	1.4	1.4
Spaghetti with Sausages in Tomato Sauce	Heinz	82.0	3.7	11.0	2.6	0.5

Spanish Chicken Tonight Sauce	Batchelors	44.0	1.7	5.8	1.5	1.3
Spanish Paella Snackpot as sold	Findus Lean Cuisine	115	4.8	17.0	3.2	0.8
Spanish Rices of the World	Batchelors	360	9.5	75.5	2.2	2.5
Rib 'n' Saucy Nik Naks, per pack	Golden Wonder	185	1.7	18.9	11.4	0.4
Spearmint Chewing Gum	Wrigley	281	nil	N	nil	nil
Special K		377	15.3	81.7	1.0	2.0
	Kellogg's	370	15.0	75.0	1.0	2.5
Special Rice Mix	Ross	59.0	2.6	13.5	0.4	2.0
Special Vegetable Mix	Ross	46.0	3.0	11.2	0.3	3.5
Spiced Basmati Rice	Sharwood	365	9.3	73.2	1.7	nil
Spiced Fruit Chutney	Baxters	143	0.6	34.8	0.1	0.8
Spiced Poppadums	Sharwood	281	20.4	45.6	1.9	10.3

All amounts given per 100g/100ml unless otherwise stated

Product	Brand	Calories kcal	Protein (g)	Carbo-hydrate (g)	Fat (g)	Dietary Fibre (g)
Spicy Arrabbiata Premium Pasta Sauce	Napolina	62.0	1.3	7.2	3.1	0.9
Spicy Beef Stew	Tyne Brand	106	7.5	8.1	5.1	n/a
Spicy Chicken Filler	Primula	242	9.0	6.0	20.3	1.0
Spicy Chicken Mexican Sauce	Homepride	80.0	1.0	17.0	0.7	n/a
Spicy Curry Pot Noodle	Golden Wonder	426	11.5	59.3	15.8	3.5
Spicy Lasagne	Findus Red Box	85.0	4.9	11.2	2.3	0.7
Spicy Lattice Fries	McCain	183	2.6	22.8	9.0	n/a
Spicy Mayhem Barbecue Sauce	HP	156	0.9	36.7	Tr	n/a
Spicy Mexican Chicken	Birds Eye	247	14.6	16.5	13.6	0.6
Spicy Mexican Dip	Primula	324	4.7	4.8	31.7	n/a
Spicy Parsnip Soup	Baxters	40.0	1.0	8.5	0.5	0.3
Spicy Pepperoni Pasta	Heinz	83.0	2.9	9.1	3.9	0.5

Spicy Prawn 3 Minute Noodles	Crosse & Blackwell	335	14.2	65.5	1.6	2.9
Spicy Salsa Twists	Heinz	75.0	2.7	10.9	2.3	0.8
Spicy Sausage & Herb Dry Mix, as sold	Crosse & Blackwell	280	7.1	49.0	5.9	2.1
Spicy Thai Chicken Soup	Baxters	67.0	1.8	7.1	3.5	0.3
Spicy Tomato & Pepperoni Pasta Bake	Homepride	72.0	1.5	8.1	3.7	n/a
Spicy Tomato & Rice with Sweetcorn Soup	Baxters	45.0	1.3	9.2	0.3	0.6
Spicy Tomato Cup-A-Soup, per sachet	Batchelors	76.0	1.8	15.5	0.8	0.8
Spicy Tomato Pizza Topping	Napolina	66.0	1.6	9.0	2.6	1.0
Spicy Tomato Salsa Pot Noodle	Golden Wonder	429	11.5	61.6	15.2	3.2
Spicy Tomato Wheat Crunchies, per pack	Golden Wonder	171	3.8	19.4	8.7	1.0

All amounts given per 100g/100ml unless otherwise stated

Product	*Brand*	*Calories kcal*	*Protein (g)*	*Carbo-hydrate (g)*	*Fat (g)*	*Dietary Fibre (g)*
Spicy Tortellini Italiana	Heinz Weight Watchers	60.0	2.8	9.9	1.0	0.9
Spicy Vegetable with Noodle Cup-A- Soup Extra, per sachet	Batchelors	111	2.8	22.0	1.3	1.8
Spicy Wedge Fries	McCain	157	2.7	24.8	5.2	n/a
Spinach, raw		25.0	2.8	1.6	0.8	2.1
boiled		19.0	2.2	0.8	0.8	2.1
frozen, boiled		21.0	3.1	0.5	0.8	2.1
Spinach & Lentil Spread, per pack	Boots Shapers	87.0	n/a	n/a	3.2	n/a
Spirits, 40% volume (mean of brandy, gin, rum, vodka, whisky)		222	Tr	Tr	nil	nil
Split Pea & Lentil Soup	Heinz Weight Watchers	32.0	1.6	6.0	0.2	0.6
Split Peas, dried, boiled		126	8.3	22.7	0.9	2.7

Food	Brand					
Sponge Cake		459	6.4	52.4	26.3	0.9
fatless		294	10.1	53.0	6.1	0.9
jam filled		302	4.2	64.2	4.9	1.8
with butter icing		490	4.5	52.4	30.6	0.6
Sponge Cake Mixes: *see individual flavours*						
Sponge Pudding		340	5.8	45.3	16.3	1.1
Sport Biscuits	McVitie's	516	6.4	62.9	26.5	1.7
Spotted Dick	McVitie's	357	5.7	51.2	15.0	2.3
Spreads, Dairy, Low Fat, etc.: *see individual brands/flavours*						
Spring Greens, raw		33.0	3.0	3.1	1.0	3.4
boiled		20.0	1.9	1.6	0.7	0.7
Spring Onion Crisps, per pack	Golden Wonder	131	1.5	12.3	8.4	1.1
Spring Onions, bulbs & tops, raw		23.0	2.0	3.0	0.5	1.5
Spring Vegetable Soup	Campbell's	21.0	0.4	4.6	Tr	n/a
	Heinz	31.0	0.8	6.2	0.4	0.7

All amounts given per 100g/100ml unless otherwise stated

Product	*Brand*	*Calories kcal*	*Protein (g)*	*Carbo-hydrate (g)*	*Fat (g)*	*Dietary Fibre (g)*
Sprouts: ***see Brussels Sprouts***						
Spry Crisp 'n' Dry, solid/oil	Van den Bergh	900	nil	nil	100	n/a
Square Cut White Bread	Hovis	234	9.5	44.3	2.1	2.4
Squash: ***see Courgettes***						
Standard Pizza Bases	Napolina	298	8.5	56.0	4.4	n/a
Starbar	Cadbury	440	9.1	55.0	31.6	n/a
Starburst	Mars	411	0.3	85.3	7.6	n/a
Starburst Joosters	Mars	356	0.0	88.8	0.1	n/a
Starburst Orange and Lemon	Mars	119	0.2	29.3	0.1	n/a
Starburst Strawberry	Mars	124	0.1	30.7	0.1	n/a
Starburst Tropical	Mars	120	0.3	29.6	0.1	n/a
Star Wars	Cadbury	550	7.0	53.7	34.1	n/a
Steak: ***see Beef***						

Steak & Kidney Pie, individual		323	9.1	25.6	21.2	0.9
	Ross	232	8.5	22.4	12.4	0.9
pastry top only		286	15.2	15.9	18.4	0.6
Steak & Onion Crisps, per pack	Golden Wonder	179	2.1	16.7	11.6	1.4
Steak in Red Wine Platter, per meal	Birds Eye Healthy Options	335	27.0	37.0	8.4	3.2
Stem Ginger Cookies	Heinz Weight Watchers	399	5.0	64.5	13.4	1.4
Stew: ***see individual flavours***						
Stewed Steak with Gravy, canned		176	14.8	1.0	1.25	Tr
Sticky Toffee Sponge Pudding	Heinz	313	3.2	46.9	12.5	0.7
Stilton, blue		411	22.7	0.1	35.5	nil
Stir Fry Chinese Style Rice	Uncle Ben's	143	2.7	26.3	3.0	n/a
Stir Fry Noodles	Sharwood	358	7.3	79.6	1.2	3.7
Stock Cubes: ***see individual flavours***						

All amounts given per 100g/100ml unless otherwise stated

Product	*Brand*	*Calories kcal*	*Protein (g)*	*Carbo-hydrate (g)*	*Fat (g)*	*Dietary Fibre (g)*
Stollen Slices	Mr Kipling	355	5.0	52.2	13.3	n/a
Stone Baked Pizza Bases	Napolina	274	8.5	55.0	2.2	n/a
Stork Margarine block	Van den Bergh	720	Tr	0.1	80.0	nil
Stork Margarine tub	Van den Bergh	658	0.1	0.1	73.0	nil
Stout, bottled		37.0	0.3	4.2	Tr	nil
extra		39.0	0.3	2.1	Tr	nil
Straight Cut Chips	McCain	127	2.8	23.0	2.6	n/a
Straight Micro Chips	McCain	207	3.5	24.7	10.5	n/a
Strawberries, raw		27.0	0.8	6.0	0.1	1.1
canned in syrup		65.0	0.5	16.9	Tr	0.7
Strawberry & Cream Cheesecake	Young's	296	4.6	31.9	16.9	0.2
Strawberry & Cream Mivi, each	Lyons Maid	83.0	1.0	13.4	2.7	n/a

Strawberry & Vanilla Sundae, per pack	Boots Shapers	121	n/a	n/a	4.2	n/a
Strawberry Bio Splitpot, per pack	Boots Shapers	79.0	n/a	n/a	0.2	n/a
Strawberry Bio Yogurt	Holland & Barrett	54.0	4.4	5.6	1.5	nil
	St Ivel	65.0	5.2	7.6	1.1	0.1
Strawberry Blancmange Powder, as sold	Brown & Polson	342	0.6	83.0	0.7	n/a
Strawberry Bonbons	Trebor Bassett	415	1.0	85.5	7.5	nil
Strawberry Cheesecake	Green's	258	3.0	31.5	12.0	n/a
	Heinz Weight Watchers	159	5.9	24.0	4.1	0.4
	McVitie's	390	4.9	31.9	22.7	0.4
Strawberry Chewits	Leaf	392	0.4	90.8	3.0	nil
Strawberry Country Crisp	Jordans	442	7.3	65.8	16.6	6.9
Strawberry Cream Cake	McVitie's	271	3.2	37.4	12.8	1.6

All amounts given per 100g/100ml unless otherwise stated

Product	*Brand*	*Calories kcal*	*Protein (g)*	*Carbo-hydrate (g)*	*Fat (g)*	*Dietary Fibre (g)*
Strawberry Creme de Creme, each	Lyons Maid	174	2.3	26.0	7.2	n/a
Strawberry Crisp	Mornflake	439	6.8	69.5	14.8	3.8
Strawberry Crusha	Burgess	101	Tr	24.6	nil	nil
Strawberry Custard Yogurt	Boots Shapers	51.0	n/a	n/a	0.8	n/a
Strawberry Dessert Mouse	St Ivel Shape	57.0	3.7	4.3	2.3	0.1
Strawberry Delight	Boots Shapers	90.0	n/a	n/a	2.5	n/a
Strawberry Flavour Custard Dessert	Ambrosia	99.0	2.7	16.3	2.6	0.1
Strawberry Flavour Jelly Crystals	Dietade	7.0	1.5	0.1	nil	nil
Strawberry Fromage Frais	St Ivel Shape	69.0	6.9	6.9	1.2	Tr
	Ski	123	6.1	14.0	4.8	n/a
Strawberry Fruit Spread	Heinz Weight Watchers	115	0.2	28.4	nil	0.4

Strawberry Fruit Sundae, per pack	Boots Shapers	80.0	n/a	n/a	4.0	n/a
Strawberry Gateau	McVitie's	274	2.3	30.4	16.4	1.0
Strawberry Heaven Dessert	St Ivel Shape	110	1.9	22.7	1.3	1.3
Strawberry Hot 'n' Fruity Custard Pots, each	Bird's	173	1.7	32.5	4.1	0.1
Strawberry Ice Cream	Fiesta	176	3.8	18.5	10.2	n/a
	Lyons Maid	84.0	1.7	10.5	3.8	n/a
per pack	Boots Shapers	102	n/a	n/a	3.9	n/a
Strawberry Ice Dessert	Provamel	103	1.2	10.7	6.2	nil
Strawberry Jam, sucrose free	Dietade	257	0.3	63.8	Tr	n/a
Strawberry Jam Mini Rolls	Cadbury	393	4.8	56.1	15.9	n/a
Strawberry Jam Sponge Pudding	Heinz	282	2.7	51.2	7.4	0.6
Strawberry Jelly, ready to eat	Rowntree	67.0	0.1	16.7	Tr	0.5
Strawberry King Cone, each	Lyons Maid	186	2.0	28.9	6.8	n/a

All amounts given per 100g/100ml unless otherwise stated

Product	*Brand*	*Calories kcal*	*Protein (g)*	*Carbo-hydrate (g)*	*Fat (g)*	*Dietary Fibre (g)*
Strawberry Luxury Trifle	St Ivel	166	2.0	21.7	7.9	0.2
Strawberry Mousse, each	Fiesta	75.0	1.7	9.0	3.6	n/a
Strawberry Mr Men, each	Lyons Maid	28.0	nil	7.0	nil	n/a
Strawberry Napoli	Lyons Maid	102	1.8	12.2	5.1	n/a
Strawberry Nesquik	Nestlé	390	nil	96.7	0.5	nil
made up with whole milk	Nestlé	168	6.8	18.8	7.8	n/a
with semi-skimmed milk	Nestlé	155	6.8	24.8	3.4	nil
ready to drink	Nestlé	68.0	3.2	10.2	1.6	nil
Strawberry Nesquik Dessert	Nestlé	445	3.5	75.8	14.3	0.3
Strawberry Pavlova	McVitie's	330	2.3	32.7	21.1	nil
Strawberry Preserve	Baxters	210	Tr	53.0	Tr	0.5
Strawberry Rice Dessert	St Ivel	121	2.8	21.3	2.7	0.1
	St Ivel Shape	77.0	3.0	14.3	0.9	0.5
Strawberry Sundaes	Mr Kipling	361	2.7	54.2	14.8	n/a

Strawberry Surprise Hot Chocolate, per pack	Boots Shapers	40.0	n/a	n/a	0.9	n/a
Strawberry Trifle	St Ivel	172	2.4	21.0	8.7	0.2
	Young's	142	1.4	26.6	3.7	0.2
Strawberry Twinpot Yogurt	St Ivel Shape	52.0	4.6	7.3	0.1	0.1
Strawberry Yogurt fat free, as sold	Boots Shapers	83.0	n/a	n/a	0.1	n/a
	St Ivel Shape	56.0	5.3	7.3	0.2	0.1
Strawberry Yogurt Mousse, as sold	Boots Shapers	89..0	n/a	n/a	3.5	n/a
Straw Mushroom: *see Mushrooms*						
Stringfellows Oven Chips	McCain	164	2.3	23.2	6.9	n/a
Strong Ale		72.0	0.7	6.1	Tr	nil
Stuffed Pork Roll	Tyne Brand	147	4.5	9.6	7.0	n/a
Stuffed Turkey Roll	Tyne Brand	150	13.0	7.8	7.4	n/a

All amounts given per 100g/100ml unless otherwise stated

Product	Brand	Calories kcal	Protein (g)	Carbo-hydrate (g)	Fat (g)	Dietary Fibre (g)
Stuffing Mixes: ***see individual flavours***						
Suet, shredded		826	Tr	12.1	86.7	0.5
Sugar: ***see Caster, Granulated, etc.***						
Sugar Puffs		324	5.9	84.5	0.8	3.2
	Quaker	387	6.5	86.5	1.0	3.0
Sugared Almonds	Cravens	430	4.4	78.1	11.1	2.3
Sultana & Apple Crunch	Mornflake	408	9.7	64.8	12.2	6.6
Sultana & Cinnamon Cookies	Heinz Weight Watchers	398	5.0	67.1	12.1	1.8
Sultana & Syrup Pancakes	Sunblest	272	5.9	51.7	4.6	1.4
Sultana Bran		303	8.5	67.8	1.6	10.0
	Kellogg's	320	9.0	66.0	2.0	13.0
Sultanas		275	2.7	69.4	0.4	2.0
	Holland & Barrett	292	2.7	69.4	0.4	2.0

Summer Fruit Layered Dessert, per pack	Boots Shapers	90.0	n/a	n/a	2.4	n/a
Summer Fruit Shorties	Jacob's Vitalinea	431	6.1	74.1	12.2	1.9
Summer Fruits Special R	Robinsons	9.6	0.1	1.2	Tr	n/a
Summer Fruits Torte	St Ivel Shape	107	2.7	20.0	1.7	1.4
Summer Fruits with Custard Twinpot Yogurt	St Ivel Shape	49.0	4.7	6.6	0.1	0.2
Sunblest Bread, etc.: *see individual flavours*						
Sundried Tomato & Herb Savoury Snack	Jordans	406	6.5	70.7	10.8	3.3
Sunflower Seed Oil		899	Tr	nil	99.9	nil
Sunflower Seeds	Holland & Barrett	596	23.4	18.6	47.5	6.0
Sunflower Spread	Vitalite	685	0.2	1.3	75.0	nil
reduced fat	Vitalite	510	0.2	1.3	56.0	nil

All amounts given per 100g/100ml unless otherwise stated

Product	*Brand*	*Calories kcal*	*Protein (g)*	*Carbo-hydrate (g)*	*Fat (g)*	*Dietary Fibre (g)*
Sunfruit Juice, per pack	Boots Shapers	41.0	n/a	n/a	Tr	n/a
Sunmalt Malt Loaf	Sunblest	286	8.6	60.3	1.1	3.7
Super Chicken Cup Soup	Knorr	326	10.4	62.6	3.8	0.7
Super Chicken Noodle Real Soup in Seconds	Knorr	296	16.3	47.6	4.5	0.3
Super Chicken Noodle Soup	Knorr	325	12.9	57.8	4.7	1.9
Super Deluxe SGFY Pizza	McCain	167	10.7	25.9	3.6	n/a
Superfast Oats	Mornflake	364	11.8	62.0	7.6	7.2
Supernoodles (Batchelors): *see individual flavours*						
Super Value Vanilla Ice Cream	Fiesta	154	3.4	20.4	7.1	n/a
Sustain	Kellogg's	360	9.0	74.0	3.5	6.0
Swede, boiled		11.0	0.3	2.3	0.1	0.7
Swedish Cauliflower & Broccoli Soups of the World	Knorr	458	6.5	43.9	28.5	3.4

Sweet & Sour Barbecue Sauce	Heinz	125	1.0	26.3	1.7	0.4
Sweet & Sour Chicken	Vesta	108	2.8	22.8	1.2	n/a
per single serving	Vesta	525	14.2	104.3	5.7	n/a
Sweet & Sour Chicken Platter, each	Birds Eye Healthy Options	410	28.0	56.0	8.0	3.4
Sweet & Sour Cook-In-Sauce	Homepride	99.0	0.4	24.4	0.1	n/a
Sweet & Sour King Prawns	Ross	195	6.6	15.1	12.2	0.4
Sweet & Sour Pork Stir Fry Dry Mix, as sold	Crosse & Blackwell	385	2.8	84.1	3.2	0.6
Sweet & Sour Pot Noodle	Golden Wonder	435	11.7	57.9	17.3	3.7
Sweet & Sour Sauce	Amoy	171	Tr	33.7	3.9	n/a
Straight to Wok	Amoy	186	0.3	45.5	0.3	n/a
	Burgess	150	0.6	35.2	Tr	0.2
Sweet & Sour Sauce & Vegetable Stir Fry	Uncle Ben's	94.0	0.4	23.2	Tr	n/a
Sweet 'n' Sour Sauce Mix, dry, as sold	Colman's	334	3.4	78.0	0.1	n/a

All amounts given per 100g/100ml unless otherwise stated

Product	*Brand*	*Calories kcal*	*Protein (g)*	*Carbo-hydrate (g)*	*Fat (g)*	*Dietary Fibre (g)*
Sweet and Sour Sizzle & Stir Sauce	Batchelors	149	0.6	19.5	7.7	1.6
Sweet & Sour Stir Fry Sauce	Sharwood	84.0	0.6	19.9	2.2	1.1
	Uncle Ben's	104	0.3	25.7	Tr	n/a
Sweet & Sour Supernoodles	Batchelors	478	9.2	64.0	20.7	3.3
Sweetbread, lamb, fried		230	19.4	5.6	14.6	0.1
Sweet Chilli Chinese Pouring Sauce	Sharwood	187	0.6	44.4	0.8	1.5
Sweetcorn						
baby, fresh/frozen, boiled		24.0	2.5	2.7	0.4	2.0
baby, canned		23.0	2.9	2.0	0.4	1.5
kernels, boiled		111	4.2	19.6	2.3	2.2
kernels, canned		122	2.9	26.6	1.2	1.4
on-the-cob, boiled		66.0	2.5	11.6	1.4	1.3
Sweetcorn & Peppers Savoury Rice	Batchelors	360	9.9	75.3	2.1	2.2

Sweet Peanuts	Trebor Bassett	426	3.1	80.0	10.3	1.4
Sweet Pickle	Burgess	167	1.0	39.3	Tr	2.0
Sweet Potato, boiled		84.0	1.1	20.5	0.3	2.3
Swiss Gateau	Cadbury	408	5.4	54.0	18.1	n/a
Swiss Rolls, Chocolate, individual		337	4.3	58.1	11.3	N
Syrup, Golden		298	0.3	79.0	nil	nil
Szechuan Chilli Sauce & Vegetable Stir Fry	Uncle Ben's	88.0	1.2	11.1	4.4	n/a

All amounts given per 100g/100ml unless otherwise stated

T

Product	*Brand*	*Calories kcal*	*Protein (g)*	*Carbo-hydrate (g)*	*Fat (g)*	*Dietary Fibre (g)*
Table Water Biscuits	McVitie's	436	9.3	76.7	9.1	3.2
Tagliatelle Bianche, as sold	Dolmio	291	10.9	56.7	2.3	n/a
Tagliatelle Carbonara	Heinz Weight Watchers	88.0	5.3	12.2	2.0	0.4
Tagliatelle Garlic & Herbs, as sold	Dolmio	294	11.7	51.9	4.4	n/a
Tahini Paste		607	18.5	0.9	58.9	8.0

All amounts given per 100g/100ml unless otherwise stated

Product	*Brand*	*Calories kcal*	*Protein (g)*	*Carbo-hydrate (g)*	*Fat (g)*	*Dietary Fibre (g)*
Tandoori Chicken Marinade	Birds Eye	187	14.2	6.7	11.5	0.4
Tandoori Chicken with Fresh Coriander Sandwiches, per pack	Boots Shapers	193	n/a	n/a	n/a	n/a
Tandoori Curry Paste	Sharwood	237	5.0	9.1	20.1	4.7
Tandoori Curry Sauce Mix	Sharwood	221	9.5	30.1	7.0	11.1
Tandoori Marinade	Lea & Perrins	133	1.4	31.7	0.7	n/a
Tandoori Rices of the World	Batchelors	367	10.1	75.3	2.8	2.3
Tangerines, flesh only		35.0	1.0	18.0	1.5	1.3
Tangy Citrus Frusli Bar, each	Jordans	393	4.1	70.4	10.5	4.3
Tangy Lemon Corner House Cake	Lyons Cakes	413	3.7	52.4	19.1	n/a
Tangy Lemon Tartlets	Mr Kipling	389	3.5	55.2	16.6	n/a
Tangy Sandwich Pickle	Heinz Speciality	133	0.9	31.8	0.2	1.1

Tangy Tomato Pickle	Heinz Speciality	106	2.3	23.5	0.3	1.8
Tangy Tomato Spread	Primula	259	15.2	2.2	21.0	n/a
Tangy Tomato with Pasta Cup-A-Soup Extra, per sachet	Batchelors	132	3.6	24.3	2.4	2.3
Taramasalata		446	3.2	4.1	46.4	N
Tartare Sauce	Baxters	515	1.0	8.0	53.3	0.3
	Burgess	268	1.5	18.7	20.0	0.7
	Colman's	263	1.1	14.0	21.7	n/a
Taz	Cadbury	490	5.1	61.9	24.6	n/a
Teacakes	Tunnock's	413	5.2	61.0	18.1	n/a
Teacakes, toasted		329	8.9	58.3	8.3	N
Temptingly Toffee & Apricot Twinpot Yogurt	St Ivel Shape	60.0	4.4	8.5	0.1	0.2
Tequila Sunrise, per pack	Boots Shapers	47.0	n/a	n/a	nil	n/a
Teriyaki Stir Fry Sauce	Sharwood	91.0	0.9	19.7	1.0	0.3

All amounts given per 100g/100ml unless otherwise stated

Product	*Brand*	*Calories kcal*	*Protein (g)*	*Carbo-hydrate (g)*	*Fat (g)*	*Dietary Fibre (g)*
Terry's Chocolate Orange Mousse Mix	Bird's	430	6.5	64.5	16.0	1.8
Texas Griddlers, each	Birds Eye	160	12.0	5.4	9.9	0.2
Texas Hot Barbecue Sauce	Heinz	121	1.3	27.9	0.4	0.4
Thai Chicken & Lemon Grass Soups of the World	Knorr	333	9.0	63.6	4.7	2.4
Thai Coconut, Corriander & Lime Marinade	Lea & Perrins	159	1.3	25.7	6.1	n/a
Thai Curry Sauce & Vegetables Stir Fry	Uncle Ben's	91.0	1.3	11.7	4.4	n/a
Thai Hot Curry Paste	Sharwood	222	5.4	11.2	17.3	5.5
Thai Red Curry Sizzle & Stir Sauce	Batchelors	180	1.5	4.5	17.3	1.7
Thai Rices of the World	Batchelors	358	9.9	75.0	2.1	2.1
Thai Sweet Chilli Sizzle & Stir Sauce	Batchelors	136	0.6	7.5	11.4	2.9

Thick Beef & Vegetable Soup	Heinz	38.0	1.6	6.1	0.8	0.6
Thick Beef Broth	Heinz	48.0	1.7	6.9	1.5	0.4
Thick Country Vegetable with Ham Soup	Heinz	64.0	3.0	8.2	2.0	1.0
Thick Pea &Ham Soup	Heinz	51.0	3.2	8.7	0.4	1.0
Thick Potato & Leek Soup	Heinz	34.0	0.7	6.5	0.6	0.5
Thick Scotch Broth	Heinz	47.0	2.1	8.1	0.7	0.9
Thomas the Tank Engine Pasta Shapes	Heinz	62.0	2.1	12.6	0.4	0.7
Thousand Island Dressing	Kraft	365	0.9	19.0	31.5	0.4
fat free	Kraft	90.0	0.5	20.5	0.2	2.8
Thousand Island Prawnnaise	Lyons Seafoods	405	6.3	3.0	41.6	n/a
Thread Noodles	Amoy	169	6.0	24.5	5.2	n/a
	Sharwood	322	11.5	69.2	1.9	3.4
Three Wishes	Cadbury	520	6.8	58.5	28.8	n/a
Tiger King Prawns, cooked	Lyons Seafoods	61.0	13.5	nil	0.6	n/a

All amounts given per 100g/100ml unless otherwise stated

Product	*Brand*	*Calories kcal*	*Protein (g)*	*Carbo-hydrate (g)*	*Fat (g)*	*Dietary Fibre (g)*
Tiger Prawns, headless + shell	Lyons Seafoods	84.0	19.6	nil	0.7	n/a
Tikka Curry Paste	Sharwood	163	3.9	7.6	13.0	4.2
Tikka 'Marinade in Minutes'	Knorr	288	4.7	59.2	3.6	n/a
Tikka Masala Classic Curry Sauce	Homepride	89.0	1.7	13.7	6.0	n/a
Tikka Masala Curry Sauce	Sharwood	99.0	3.0	8.4	5.8	2.3
Tikka Masala Low in Fat Sauce	Homepride	55.0	1.2	11.0	1.1	n/a
Tikka Masala Sizzle & Stir Sauce	Batchelors	200	2.0	8.4	17.6	2.6
Tikka 95% Fat Free Dip	St Ivel Shape	90.0	7.6	6.6	3.7	0.1
Tikka Prawnnaise Light	Lyons Seafoods	218	5.2	6.1	19.3	n/a
Tikka Soured Cream Dip	St Ivel	391	2.6	5.2	40.0	0.1
Time Out	Cadbury	555	5.0	59.4	32.9	n/a
Time Out Orange	Cadbury	555	5.0	59.4	32.9	n/a

Tip Top	Nestlé	112	4.8	9.0	6.3	nil
Tiramisu	McVitie's	337	3.5	31.2	22.2	0.3
Tizer	Barr	39.0	Tr	9.6	Tr	nil
Toast: ***see Bread***						
Toasted Crunchy Oatbran	Mornflake	350	16.5	53.5	7.8	14.6
Toasted Oat Crunchy with vine fruits and malt	Mornflake	411	11.0	87.0	11.0	7.0
Toasted Sesame Pitta Bread	International Harvest	263	9.7	48.0	3.6	3.0
Toast Toppers (Heinz): ***see individual flavours***						
Toffee Bonbons	Trebor Bassett	430	1.4	81.7	10.8	nil
Toffee Cheesecake	Green's	342	3.2	37.5	19.3	n/a
Toffee Chocolate Dessert	Heinz Weight Watchers	190	5.9	32.9	3.6	0.4
Toffee Crisp	Nestlé Rowntree	494	4.1	62.1	25.5	0.5

All amounts given per 100g/100ml unless otherwise stated

Product	*Brand*	*Calories kcal*	*Protein (g)*	*Carbo-hydrate (g)*	*Fat (g)*	*Dietary Fibre (g)*
Toffee Crisp Dessert Split Pot	Chambourcy	225	4.0	27.1	11.0	n/a
Toffee Crumble, each	Lyons Maid	170	1.9	19.6	9.3	n/a
Toffee Flavour Custard Dessert	Ambrosia	100	2.7	16.5	2.6	0.1
Toffee Flavour & Toffee Sauce Iced Dessert	Heinz Weight Watchers	163	2.7	26.2	4.8	0.2
Toffee Flavour Fudge Swirl Iced Dessert	Heinz Weight Watchers	143	2.5	22.6	4.4	0.4
Toffee Mousse, each	Fiesta	78.0	1.8	9.6	3.8	n/a
Toffee Napoli	Lyons Maid	107	1.8	14.5	5.8	n/a
Toffees, mixed		430	2.1	71.1	17.2	nil
Toffee YoYo	McVitie's	476	5.3	66.9	20.9	1.0
Toffo	Nestlé Rowntree	452	2.2	69.9	18.2	n/a

Tofu (soya bean curd)						
steamed		73.0	8.1	0.7	4.2	N
steamed, fried		261	23.5	2.0	17.7	N
Tomato & Bacon Pasta 'n' Sauce	Batchelors	355	13.0	70.0	2.6	3.7
Tomato & Basil Pasta Choice Mix, as sold	Crosse & Blackwell	370	12.3	70.3	3.9	3.1
Tomato & Brown Lentil Soup	Baxters	39.0	2.4	8.7	0.1	1.5
Tomato & Herb Delicately Flavoured Rice	Batchelors	387	7.8	79.4	4.2	5.0
Tomato & Herb Potato Bake	Homepride	191	2.0	4.9	18.2	n/a
Tomato & Lentil Slim-A-Soup, per sachet	Batchelors	57.0	2.5	10.9	0.3	1.6
Tomato & Lentil Soup	Heinz	54.0	2.7	10.4	0.2	1.0
Tomato & Herb Marinade	Lea & Perrins	100	1.2	24.1	0.5	n/a
Tomato & Mozzarella Tastebreaks Pasta Snacks	Knorr	402	11.7	60.5	12.6	n/a

All amounts given per 100g/100ml unless otherwise stated

Product	*Brand*	*Calories kcal*	*Protein (g)*	*Carbo-hydrate (g)*	*Fat (g)*	*Dietary Fibre (g)*
Tomato & Onion Cook-In-Sauce	Homepride	47.0	0.9	9.8	0.5	n/a
Tomato & Orange Soup	Baxters	40.0	1.0	8.5	0.5	0.3
Tomato & Prawn Premium Pasta Sauce	Napolina	76.0	3.0	8.0	3.5	0.5
Tomato & Sausage Bronto's Monster Feet	McVitie's	208	8.4	28.9	7.3	n/a
Tomato & Tarragon Low In Fat Sauce	Homepride	43.0	1.0	7.6	1.3	n/a
Tomato & Vegetable Cup-A-Soup, per sachet	Batchelors	107	2.4	18.6	2.6	1.3
Tomato & Vegetable Soup, per pack	Boots Shapers	37.0	n/a	n/a	0.6	n/a
Tomato & Vegetable Soup, organic	Baxters	33.0	0.9	6.6	0.3	0.6
Tomato Chutney		161	1.2	40.9	0.4	1.4

Tomato Cup-A-Soup, per sachet	Batchelors	85.0	0.8	17.3	1.4	1.2
Tomatoes, raw		17.0	0.7	3.1	0.3	1.0
fried in oil		91.0	0.7	5.0	7.7	1.3
grilled		49.0	2.0	8.9	0.9	2.9
canned		16.0	1.0	3.0	0.1	0.7
cherry, raw		18.0	0.8	3.0	0.4	1.0
Tomato Frito	Heinz	73.0	1.3	7.7	4.1	0.8
Tomato Juice		14.0	0.8	3.0	Tr	0.6
	Del Monte	19.0	0.8	3.5	Tr	n/a
	Napolina	16.0	0.7	3.4	Tr	n/a
Tomato Juice Cocktail	Britvic	20.0	0.9	3.5	0.1	n/a
Tomato Ketchup		98.0	2.1	24.0	Tr	0.9
	Crosse & Blackwell	125	1.0	28.2	0.1	0.2
	Daddies	110	0.9	26.5	0.3	n/a
	Heinz	107	1.0	24.7	0.1	0.6
Tomato Lasagne Sauce	Ragu	37.0	1.5	7.4	0.2	1.0

All amounts given per 100g/100ml unless otherwise stated

Product	*Brand*	*Calories kcal*	*Protein (g)*	*Carbo-hydrate (g)*	*Fat (g)*	*Dietary Fibre (g)*
Tomato, Onion & Herb Pasta 'n' Sauce	Batchelors	348	13.2	64.5	4.1	5.8
Tomato Puree		68.0	4.5	12.9	0.2	2.8
	Napolina	90.0	4.8	18.0	Tr	n/a
Tomato Cup Soup	Knorr	335	11.7	47.6	10.9	5.5
Tomato Rice Soup	Campbell's	46.0	0.9	8.3	1.0	n/a
Tomato, Salmon & Marscarpone Premium Pasta Sauce	Napolina	95.0	3.1	8.5	5.4	0.6
Tomato Sauce		89.0	2.2	8.6	5.5	1.4
	Burgess	156	1.3	34.4	0.8	0.7
Tomato Sauce Crisps, per pack	Golden Wonder	130	1.4	12.3	8.4	1.1
Tomato Scooples	Kavli	352	11.5	75.6	2.5	4.5
Tomato Soup, dried, as served		31.0	0.6	6.3	0.5	N
dried, as sold		321	6.6	65.0	5.6	N

low calorie	Heinz Weight Watchers	26.0	0.7	4.7	0.5	0.3
Tomato with Red Pepper Chutney	Baxters	164	2.0	38.0	0.4	1.5
Tongue, canned		213	16.0	nil	16.5	nil
Tonic Water	Schweppes	21.8	nil	5.1	nil	n/a
Topic	Mars	497	7.4	56.7	26.7	n/a
TOPS Chocolate Flavour Syrup	Tate & Lyle	305	1.0	74.0	0.5	nil
TOPS Maple Flavour Syrup	Tate & Lyle	306	Tr	76.5	nil	nil
TOPS Strawberry Flavour Syrup	Tate & Lyle	308	Tr	77.5	nil	nil
TOPS Toffee Flavour Syrup	Tate & Lyle	306	Tr	76.5	nil	nil
Tornado, each	Lyons Maid	61.0	nil	15.2	nil	n/a
Tortellini Italiana	Heinz Weight Watchers	62.0	2.0	9.4	1.8	0.6

All amounts given per 100g/100ml unless otherwise stated

Product	*Brand*	*Calories kcal*	*Protein (g)*	*Carbo-hydrate (g)*	*Fat (g)*	*Dietary Fibre (g)*
Tortelloni 5 Cheese, as sold	Dolmio	334	14.7	44.6	10.7	n/a
Tortelloni Italian Ham, as sold	Dolmio	297	15.3	41.1	7.9	n/a
Tortelloni Mushroom & Garlic, as sold	Dolmio	275	10.3	45.2	5.8	n/a
Tortelloni Veg, Cheese, Garlic & Herbs, as sold	Dolmio	329	13.4	46.2	10.1	n/a
Tortilla Chips		459	7.6	60.1	22.6	4.9
Traditional Crunch with honey & raisins	Mornflake	418	9.5	67.2	12.3	6.8
Traditional Golden Pouring Syrup	Lyle's	308	0.4	76.0	nil	nil
Traditional Lemonade	Boots Shapes	25.0	n/a	n/a	Tr	n/a
Traditional Malt Bakes	McVitie's	502	5.9	67.0	22.9	1.8
Traditional Rice Pudding with Sultanas & Nutmeg	Ambrosia	105	3.2	16.6	2.9	0.1

Traditional Sauce for Pasta	Ragu	67.0	2.0	9.9	2.1	2.1
Traffic Jams	Lyons Cakes	359	3.7	54.7	14.0	n/a
Trail Mix		432	9.1	37.2	28.5	4.3
Treacle, black		257	1.2	67.2	nil	nil
Treacle Lattice Tart	Mr Kipling	384	4.2	63.3	12.6	n/a
Treacle Sponge Pudding	Heinz	278	2.3	49.2	8.0	0.6
Treacle Tart		368	3.7	60.4	14.1	1.1
Treasure Crunch	Mornflake	400	8.5	68.1	10.4	5.1
Trebor Mints	Trebor Bassett	399	0.6	98.0	0.4	nil
Trifle		160	3.6	22.3	6.3	0.5
Trifle Mixes, as sold	Bird's					
Chocolate & Caramel		410	3.9	74.0	11.0	1.4
Fruit Cocktail		425	2.7	78.0	11.0	1.2
Raspberry		425	2.7	78.0	10.5	1.2
Sherry Flavour		425	2.7	78.0	11.0	1.2
Strawberry		425	2.7	78.0	10.5	1.2

All amounts given per 100g/100ml unless otherwise stated

Product	*Brand*	*Calories kcal*	*Protein (g)*	*Carbo-hydrate (g)*	*Fat (g)*	*Dietary Fibre (g)*
Trifle Sponge	Lyons Cakes	323	5.3	71.9	1.5	n/a
Trifle with Fresh Cream		166	2.4	19.5	9.2	0.5
Trio Toffy	Jacob's	535	5.0	61.2	30.0	1.6
Tripe, dressed		60.0	9.4	nil	2.5	nil
dressed, stewed		100	14.8	nil	4.5	nil
Triple Chocolate Crisp	Mornflake	435	7.1	67.7	15.1	4.9
Triple X Mints	Nestlé Rowntree	393	0.7	97.6	nil	n/a
Tropical Alpen	Weetabix	367	11.0	65.1	6.9	7.8
Tropical Fruit Burst	Del Monte	45.0	0.2	10.9	Tr	n/a
Tropical Fruit Drink, per pack	Boots Shapers	nil	n/a	n/a	nil	n/a
Tropical Fruit Solar	McVitie's	456	6.1	56.5	22.9	1.8
Tropical Juice Bar, each	Lyons Maid	37.0	Tr	9.9	Tr	n/a
Tropical Mix	Ross	64.0	2.5	9.5	2.8	2.4

Tropical Original Crunchy	Jordans	425	8.5	65.8	14.2	6.2
Tropical Prawns	Lyons Seafoods	51.0	12.0	nil	0.5	n/a
cooked & peeled	Lyons Seafoods	53.0	12.0	nil	0.6	n/a
in brine	Lyons Seafoods	71.0	14.3	2.0	0.7	n/a
Tropical Special R Ready to Drink Carton	Robinsons	5.0	0.1	0.9	Tr	n/a
Tropical Squash, undiluted	St Clements	186	0.3	44.4	0.2	n/a
Trout, brown, steamed, flesh only		135	23.5	nil	4.5	nil
Tuc Biscuits	McVitie's	530	7.1	60.8	28.1	2.1
Tuc Savoury Sandwich Biscuits	McVitie's	571	8.0	49.5	37.5	1.5
Tuna						
canned in oil, drained		189	27.1	nil	9.0	nil
canned in brine, drained		99.0	23.5	nil	0.6	nil
Tuna & Mayonnaise Spread	Shippams	252	19.0	2.7	18.4	n/a
Tuna & Pasta Bake Casserole Mix, as sold	Colman's	314	11.0	54.0	4.9	n/a

All amounts given per 100g/100ml unless otherwise stated

Product	*Brand*	*Calories kcal*	*Protein (g)*	*Carbo-hydrate (g)*	*Fat (g)*	*Dietary Fibre (g)*
Tuna & Sweetcorn Filler	Primula	186	10.7	4.1	14.1	1.2
Tuna & Sweetcorn 95% Fat Free Dip	St Ivel Shape	94.0	8.7	6.2	3.8	0.1
Tuna Chunks/Steaks						
Canned in Brine	Heinz	99.0	23.5	nil	0.6	nil
Canned in Vegetable Oil	Heinz	189	27.1	nil	9.0	nil
Tuna Crumble	Ross	191	7.5	14.4	11.9	0.6
Tuna Creamy Pasta Bake	Napolina	88.0	3.1	10.6	3.7	0.4
Tuna Pasta Bake	Heinz Baked Bean Cuisine	103	6.6	12.8	2.8	1.2
Tuna, Pepper & Sweetcorn Salad with Mayonnaise Sandwich, per pack	Boots Shapers	306	20.0	34.0	10.0	5.8
Tuna Salad Sandwich	Heinz Weight Watchers	137	10.5	13.9	4.4	2.4
Tuna Sandwich Filler	Heinz	192	6.3	11.7	13.4	0.3

Tuna Twists Italiana	Heinz Weight Watchers	62.0	4.3	8.1	1.4	0.6
Tunes	Mars	392	nil	98.1	nil	n/a
Turkey, roast						
meat only		140	28.8	nil	2.7	nil
meat & skin		171	28.0	nil	6.5	nil
light meat		132	29.8	nil	1.4	nil
dark meat		148	27.8	nil	4.1	nil
Turkey & Herb Spread	Shippams	151	16.8	4.4	7.4	n/a
Turkey Casserole Classic Creations Mix, as sold	Crosse & Blackwell	305	9.3	47.8	8.5	1.5
Turkish Delight	Cadbury	365	2.0	73.3	7.2	n/a
	Boots Shapers	307	n/a	n/a	9.3	n/a
	Trebor Bassett	323	Tr	85.8	nil	Tr
Turkish Delight without nuts		295	0.6	77.9	nil	nil
Turnip, boiled		12.0	0.6	2.0	0.2	1.9
Tuscan Chicken Regional Recipe	Ragu	42.0	1.4	8.0	0.5	0.9

All amounts given per 100g/100ml unless otherwise stated

Product	*Brand*	*Calories kcal*	*Protein (g)*	*Carbo-hydrate (g)*	*Fat (g)*	*Dietary Fibre (g)*
Twiglets, Original	Jacob's	393	12.1	61.5	11.0	6.9
Tangy		448	8.3	57.8	20.4	6.0
Spicy		462	10.8	53.8	22.6	6.6
Twinpack Oatcake, per pack	Boots Shapers	n/a	n/a	n/a	3.6	n/a
Twirl	Cadbury	525	8.1	55.9	30.1	n/a
Twix	Mars	495	5.8	63.5	24.2	n/a
Twix IceCream	Mars	389	5.2	40.6	22.9	n/a
Two Fruits in Syrup	Del Monte	69.0	0.3	18.0	0.1	n/a
Tzatziki		66.0	3.7	2.0	4.9	0.2

U

Product	*Brand*	*Calories kcal*	*Protein (g)*	*Carbo-hydrate (g)*	*Fat (g)*	*Dietary Fibre (g)*
Ultra Plus Very Low Fat Cheese Spread with Herbs	Primula	137	16.0	7.0	5.0	n/a
Um Bongo Fruit Drink	Libby	43.0	Tr	10.7	Tr	Tr
Uncle Ben's Stir Fry Range: *see individual flavours*						
United Biscuits						
golden crunch	McVitie's	499	5.9	64.7	23.4	1.5
mint	McVitie's	499	5.8	67.0	23.1	1.5
orange	McVitie's	498	5.8	64.6	23.3	1.5

All amounts given per 100g/100ml unless otherwise stated

Product	*Brand*	*Calories kcal*	*Protein (g)*	*Carbo-hydrate (g)*	*Fat (g)*	*Dietary Fibre (g)*
Unsweetened Soya Milk	Holland & Barrett	36.0	3.6	0.6	2.1	1.0
Utterly Cheddarly, Crumbly	St Ivel	385	15.5	11.0	31.0	nil
Utterly Cheddarly, Smooth	St Ivel	385	15.5	11.0	31.0	nil

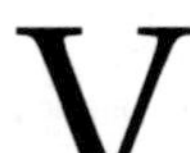

Product	*Brand*	*Calories kcal*	*Protein (g)*	*Carbo-hydrate (g)*	*Fat (g)*	*Dietary Fibre (g)*
Vanilla & Raspberry Compote Iced Dessert	Heinz Weight Watchers	142	2.6	23.3	3.9	0.3
Vanilla & Strawberry Compote Iced Dessert	Heinz Weight Watchers	142	2.5	23.4	3.9	0.2
Vanilla Blancmange Powder, as sold	Brown & Polson	341	0.6	83.0	0.7	n/a
Vanilla Creme Anglaise Sauce	Bird's	101	3.1	14.5	3.4	0.4

All amounts given per 100g/100ml unless otherwise stated

Product	*Brand*	*Calories kcal*	*Protein (g)*	*Carbo-hydrate (g)*	*Fat (g)*	*Dietary Fibre (g)*
Vanilla Creme de Creme, each	Lyons Maid	166	3.0	21.3	8.3	n/a
Vanilla Crusha	Burgess	161	nil	39.7	nil	nil
Vanilla Cup, each	Lyons Maid	181	3.3	25.5	8.1	n/a
Vanilla Dessert (in pots)	Provamel	86.0	3.0	14.4	1.8	1.0
Vanilla Flavour Dessert with Caramel Sauce	Chambourcy	108	3.3	22.8	0.8	Tr
Vanilla Flavour Custard with Coco Crunch	Ambrosia	119	3.0	20.1	3.0	0.3
Vanilla Flavour Custard with Honey Oat Crunch	Ambrosia	150	3.7	22.8	4.8	1.1
Vanilla Flavoured Soya Milk	Provamel	55.0	36.0	10.0	2.1	1.0
Vanilla Fudge	Cravens	469	1.1	77.6	17.1	nil
Vanilla Ice Cream	Fiesta	155	3.6	19.2	7.6	n/a
	Lyons Maid	87.0	1.7	11.0	4.5	n/a

Vanilla Ice Dessert	Provamel	104	1.2	10.8	6.2	nil
Vanilla Iced Dessert	Heinz Weight Watchers	124	2.4	20.1	3.5	0.2
Vanilla King Cone, each	Lyons Maid	174	2.8	23.6	7.6	n/a
Vanilla Mr Men, each	Lyons Maid	52.0	1.2	8.8	1.4	n/a
Vanilla Napoli	Lyons Maid	100	1.9	10.6	5.6	n/a
Vanilla Soft Serve Ice Cream	Fiesta	161	3.3	19.4	8.3	n/a
Vanilla Walnut Whip	Nestlé Rowntree	486	5.7	60.5	24.6	n/a
Veal						
cutlet, fried in oil		215	31.4	4.4	8.1	0.1
fillet, roast		230	31.6	nil	11.5	nil
Vegetable Bake	Ross	80.0	2.4	13.0	2.9	1.9
Vegetable Balti Mix, as sold	Crosse & Blackwell	340	12.0	45.7	12.0	5.5
Vegetable Chilli dry mix, as sold	Crosse & Blackwell	305	13.5	43.0	8.0	5.2

All amounts given per 100g/100ml unless otherwise stated

Product	*Brand*	*Calories kcal*	*Protein (g)*	*Carbo-hydrate (g)*	*Fat (g)*	*Dietary Fibre (g)*
Vegetable Curry with rice, per pack	Tyne Brand	57.0	2.0	9.6	1.4	n/a
	Birds Eye	350	7.0	57.0	10.5	2.7
Vegetable Ghee	Sharwood	897	Tr	Tr	99.7	nil
Vegetable Granules, as sold	Oxo	316	8.4	59.5	4.9	0.9
Vegetable Hotpot	Heinz Weight Watchers	68.0	2.6	9.9	1.9	1.5
Vegetable Hot Pot Dry Mix, as sold	Crosse & Blackwell	390	8.0	49.4	17.6	1.3
Vegetable Kievs	Birds Eye	155	5.2	17.2	7.2	2.0
Vegetable Lasagne dry mix, as sold	Crosse & Blackwell	440	8.2	48.2	23.8	0.9
	Heinz Weight Watchers	78.0	3.2	12.9	1.5	1.0
	Ross	110	5.3	12.6	4.7	0.9
Vegetable Oil		899	Tr	nil	99.9	nil
Vegetable Oxo Cubes, as sold	Oxo	253	11.2	41.9	4.5	1.7

Vegetable Pasta Bake Mix, as sold	Crosse & Blackwell	555	9.5	36.0	41.7	0.7
Vegetable Pie	Ross	246	5.1	27.5	13.9	2.5
Vegetable Quarter Pounders, each	Birds Eye	190	4.3	23.0	9.1	1.8
Vegetable Ravioli with Tomato Sauce Italiana	Heinz Weight Watchers	69.0	1.7	10.9	2.1	0.5
Vegetable Salad	Heinz	133	1.5	12.6	8.5	1.3
Vegetable Samosas: *see Samosas*						
Vegetable Soup, canned, ready to serve		37.0	1.5	6.7	0.7	1.5
	Campbell's	32.0	0.8	5.7	0.7	n/a
	Heinz	47.0	1.4	8.4	0.9	1.1
	Heinz Weight Watchers	31.0	1.0	5.9	0.3	0.9
Vegetable Spaghetti Bolognese, per meal	Birds Eye	275	9.8	52.0	3.2	4.3
Vegetable Stock Cubes	Knorr	308	11.9	21.7	19.3	1.3

All amounts given per 100g/100ml unless otherwise stated

Product	*Brand*	*Calories kcal*	*Protein (g)*	*Carbo-hydrate (g)*	*Fat (g)*	*Dietary Fibre (g)*
Vegetable Stroganoff	Heinz Weight Watchers	85.0	2.2	15.0	1.9	0.6
Vegetable Tuscany Bake	Birds Eye	97.0	11.8	2.2	4.6	0.6
Vegetarian Double Gloucester Cheese	Holland & Barrett	405	24.6	0.1	34.0	nil
Vegetarian Mild Cheddar Cheese	Holland & Barrett	412	25.5	0.1	34.4	nil
Vegetarian Red Leicester Cheese	Holland & Barrett	401	24.3	0.1	33.7	nil
Vegetarian Tandoori Vegetable Pasty	Holland & Barrett	188	4.4	29.9	5.7	1.8
Venison, roast, meat only		198	35.0	nil	6.4	nil
Vermouth						
dry		118	0.1	5.5	nil	nil
sweet		151	Tr	15.9	nil	nil
Very Low Fat Spread		273	8.3	3.6	25.0	nil

Vessen Pâté: ***see individual flavours***						
Victoria Sponge Mix	Green's	367	6.0	52.0	15.0	n/a
Viennese Whirls	Lyons Cakes	500	3.8	49.8	31.3	n/a
Viennese Xmas Slices	Cadbury	384	4.6	58.0	14.1	n/a
Vintage Cider: ***see Cider***						
Vintage Orange Marmalade	Baxters	252	Tr	63.0	Tr	0.8
Vitalinea (Jacob's): ***see individual products***						
Vitalite	St Ivel	578	0.4	1.2	63.0	nil
Buttery	St Ivel	638	0.9	1.0	70.0	nil
Light	St Ivel	348	1.5	Tr	38.0	nil
Vodka: ***see Spirits***						

W

Product	*Brand*	*Calories kcal*	*Protein (g)*	*Carbo-hydrate (g)*	*Fat (g)*	*Dietary Fibre (g)*
Wafer Biscuits, filled		535	4.7	66.0	29.9	N
Wafer Cream	Tunnock's	513	6.6	63.2	28.0	n/a
Waffles: *see Potato Waffles*						
Waistline Low Fat French Dressing	Crosse & Blackwell	20.0	0.2	3.2	0.2	0.1
Waistline Low Fat Vinaigrette	Crosse & Blackwell	13.0	0.7	0.4	0.1	0.2

All amounts given per 100g/100ml unless otherwise stated

Product	*Brand*	*Calories kcal*	*Protein (g)*	*Carbo-hydrate (g)*	*Fat (g)*	*Dietary Fibre (g)*
Waistline Reduced Fat Dressing	Crosse & Blackwell	120	0.9	14.3	6.2	0.4
Walnut Halves	Holland & Barrett	688	14.7	3.3	68.5	3.5
	Whitworths	525	10.6	5.0	51.5	5.2
Walnuts		688	14.7	3.3	68.5	3.5
Water Chestnuts, canned		31.0	0.9	7.4	Tr	N
	Amoy	42.0	0.9	10.1	nil	n/a
Watermelon: *see Melon*						
Weetabix	Weetabix	342	11.8	67.8	2.7	10.1
Weetaflakes	Weetabix	351	10.0	72.1	2.5	9.2
Weetos	Weetabix	385	6.3	78.8	4.9	5.5
Weight Watchers Products (Heinz): *see individual flavours*						
Wensleydale Cheese		377	23.3	0.1	31.5	nil
Wheat Flour: *see Flour, wheat*						

Wheatgerm		302	26.7	44.7	9.2	15.6
Wheatgerm Bread	Vitbe	232	10.4	39.6	3.6	4.2
Wheatgerm Oil		899	Tr	nil	99.9	nil
Whelks, boiled, weighed with shells		14.0	2.8	Tr	0.3	nil
Whisky: *see Spirits*						
Whitebait, fried		525	19.5	5.3	47.5	0.2
	Young's	96.0	15.4	nil	3.8	nil
White Bread: *see also Bread*	Heinz Weight Watchers	231	10.6	43.6	1.6	3.6
	Hovis	235	9.0	44.4	2.3	2.1
	Mothers Pride	229	8.0	45.6	1.6	3.0
	Nimble	249	10.3	46.3	2.6	2.2
	Sunblest	232	7.4	46.4	1.9	2.1
White Cap Cooking Fat	Van den Bergh	900	nil	nil	100	n/a
White Chocolate		529	8.0	58.3	30.9	nil
organic	Green & Black's	572	6.0	54.0	36.5	nil
White Chocolate Buttons	Cadbury	535	8.8	56.5	30.3	n/a

All amounts given per 100g/100ml unless otherwise stated

Product	*Brand*	*Calories kcal*	*Protein (g)*	*Carbo-hydrate (g)*	*Fat (g)*	*Dietary Fibre (g)*
White Chocolate Chip Harvest Chewy Bar, each	Quaker	94	1.3	14.5	3.3	0.7
White Custard Flavour Dessert	Ambrosia	109	2.6	19.0	2.5	0.1
White Chocolate Finger Biscuits	Cadbury	532	7.1	62.5	28.2	1.5
White Flora	Van den Bergh	900	nil	nil	100	nil
White Lasagne Sauce	Ragu	167	0.5	4.7	16.3	0.3
White Pepper: ***see Peppers***						
White Pitta Bread	International Harvest	251	8.6	50.0	1.8	2.3
White Pudding		450	7.0	36.3	31.8	N
White Rice: ***see Rice***						
White Rolls: ***see Bread Rolls***						

White Sauce						
savoury, made with whole milk		150	4.1	10.9	7.8	0.2
savoury, made with semi-skimmed milk		128	4.2	11.1	10.3	0.2
sweet, made with whole milk		170	3.8	18.6	9.5	0.2
sweet, made with semi-skimmed milk		150	3.9	18.8	7.2	0.2
White Sauce Mix, as sold	Colman's	371	11.0	58.0	9.9	n/a
White Stick, each	Nestlé	271	3.7	24.2	17.8	n/a
White Stilton Cheese: *see Stilton*						
White Wine						
dry		66.0	0.1	0.6	nil	nil
medium		75.0	0.1	3.4	nil	nil
sparkling		76.0	0.2	5.9	nil	nil
sweet		94.0	0.2	5.9	nil	nil
White Wine Cook-In-Sauce	Homepride	80.0	0.9	7.1	4.4	n/a
White Wine, Garlic & Pepper Marinade	Lea & Perrins	99.0	0.5	23.7	0.7	n/a

All amounts given per 100g/100ml unless otherwise stated

Product	*Brand*	*Calories kcal*	*Protein (g)*	*Carbo-hydrate (g)*	*Fat (g)*	*Dietary Fibre (g)*
White Wine, Mushroom & Herb Low in Fat Sauce	Homepride	40.0	0.8	7.0	1.2	n/a
Whiting						
steamed, flesh only		92.0	20.9	nil	0.9	nil
in crumbs, fried		191	18.1	7.0	10.3	0.3
Wholegrain Crispbread	Kavli	335	9.8	70.2	1.7	12.6
Wholegrain Mustard	Colman's	173	8.5	8.5	11.0	5.9
Wholegrain Mustard & Herb Potato Mashers , as sold	Colman's	510	9.7	19.1	44.1	Tr
Wholegrain Rice						
as sold	Uncle Ben's	340	8.9	70.8	2.4	n/a
frozen	Uncle Ben's	147	3.7	30.9	1.8	n/a
3 minute	Uncle Ben's	164	3.9	33.4	1.6	n/a
Wholemeal Bread	Allinson	216	9.5	39.2	2.4	6.5
organic	Allinson	217	9.5	39.6	2.3	6.5
	Nimble	216	11.2	36.9	2.7	6.9

Wholemeal Crackers		413	10.1	72.1	11.3	4.4
Wholemeal Flour: *see Flour, wholemeal*						
Wholemeal Scooples	Kavli	386	11.9	83.2	0.6	7.7
Wholemeal Light Crispbread	Allinson	349	11.7	69.7	2.6	11.0
Wholemeal Pastry: *see Pastry*						
Wholemeal Rolls, each	Allinson	151	5.5	26.6	2.5	3.7
Wholemeal Scones: *see Scones*						
Whole Milk: *see Milk*						
Wholenut Chocolate	Cadbury	550	9.3	48.8	35.2	n/a
Wholenut Tasters	Cadbury	555	9.9	44.2	37.8	n/a
Wholewheat Macaroni: *see Macaroni*						
Wholewheat Ravioli: *see Ravioli*						
Wholewheat Spaghetti: *see Spaghetti*						
Wild Berries Frusli Bar, each	Jordans	132	2.0	22.4	3.8	1.6
Wild Blackberry Jelly	Baxters	210	Tr	53.0	Tr	1.2

All amounts given per 100g/100ml unless otherwise stated

Product	*Brand*	*Calories kcal*	*Protein (g)*	*Carbo-hydrate (g)*	*Fat (g)*	*Dietary Fibre (g)*
Wildlife	Cadbury	520	7.8	56.8	29.3	n/a
Wild Rowan Jelly	Baxters	268	nil	67.0	nil	nil
Willow/Willow Lightly Salted	Dairy Crest	709	0.7	1.0	78.0	n/a
Wine: ***see Red, Rosé, White***						
Wine Gums	Trebor Bassett	337	6.0	76.7	0.1	nil
Winkles, boiled, weighed with shells		14.0	2.9	Tr	0.3	nil
Winter Vegetable Soup	Campbell's	37.0	0.7	5.0	1.6	n/a
	Heinz	46.0	2.8	8.2	0.2	1.1
	Heinz Weight Watchers	31.0	1.6	6.0	0.1	0.8
Wispa	Cadbury	550	7.1	53.9	34.2	n/a
Wispa Gold	Cadbury	515	6.2	56.2	29.7	n/a
Wispa Mint	Cadbury	550	7.0	54.7	33.6	n/a
Woodpecker Cider	H P Bulmer	30.0	n/a	n/a	n/a	n/a

Worcester Sauce Crisps, per pack	Golden Wonder	180	2.0	16.7	11.7	1.5
Worcester Sauce Wheat Crunchies, per pack	Golden Wonder	170	3.8	19.2	8.7	1.0
Worcestershire Sauce	Lea & Perrins	88.0	1.1	22.0	Tr	n/a

All amounts given per 100g/100ml unless otherwise stated

Y

Product	Brand	Calories kcal	Protein (g)	Carbo-hydrate (g)	Fat (g)	Dietary Fibre (g)
Yam, raw		114	1.5	28.2	0.3	1.3
boiled		133	1.7	33.0	0.3	1.4
Yeast, bakers, compressed		53.0	11.4	1.1	0.4	N
dried		169	35.6	3.5	1.5	N
Yellow Bean Sauce	Amoy	155	3.3	33.1	1.0	n/a
Yellow Bean Stir Fry Sauce Straight to Wok	Amoy	159	1.6	36.9	0.5	n/a
	Sharwood	129	0.3	28.9	1.7	1.5

All amounts given per 100g/100ml unless otherwise stated

Product	*Brand*	*Calories kcal*	*Protein (g)*	*Carbo-hydrate (g)*	*Fat (g)*	*Dietary Fibre (g)*
Yellow Split Peas	Whitworths	310	22.1	56.6	1.0	5.9
Yofu Black Cherry with Vanilla Non-DairyYogurt	Provamel	84.0	3.7	12.6	2.1	1.2
Yofu Natural Organic Non-Dairy Yogurt	Provamel	53.0	4.5	2.8	2.6	1.5
Yofu Peach & Mango and Red Cherry Non-Dairy Yogurt	Provamel	93.0	3.7	14.7	2.1	1.2
Yofu Strawberry with Peach Non-DairyYogurt	Provamel	90.0	4.1	12.8	2.4	1.3
Yogurt						
Greek style, cows		115	6.4	2.0	9.1	nil
Greek style, sheep		106	4.4	5.6	7.5	nil
low calorie		41.0	4.3	6.0	0.2	N
low fat, plain		56.0	5.1	7.5	0.8	N
low fat, flavoured		90.0	3.8	17.9	0.9	N
low fat, fruit		90.0	4.1	17.9	0.7	N

soya		72.0	5.0	3.9	4.2	N
whole milk, plain		79.0	5.7	7.8	3.0	N
whole milk, fruit		105	5.1	15.7	2.8	N
Yogurt & Cucumber Soured Cream Dip	St Ivel	267	3.2	4.4	26.3	0.3
Yogurt Coated Peanuts & Raisins	Holland & Barrett	490	9.7	49.8	27.5	1.7
Yorkie (Rowntree Mackintosh): ***see individual flavours***						
Yorkie Dessert	Chambourcy	215	3.9	25.3	10.8	0.7
Yorkie Dessert Split Pot	Chambourcy	250	4.1	31.6	11.5	n/a
Yorkshire Pudding		208	6.6	24.7	9.9	0.9
Young Broad Beans	Birds Eye	56.0	5.9	7.4	0.3	4.8
Young Sweetcorn	Birds Eye	93.0	2.9	18.4	0.9	1.6
Yowie	Cadbury	525	6.6	59.0	29.4	n/a
YoYo (McVitie's): ***see individual flavours***						

All amounts given per 100g/100ml unless otherwise stated

Z

Product	*Brand*	*Calories kcal*	*Protein (g)*	*Carbo-hydrate (g)*	*Fat (g)*	*Dietary Fibre (g)*
Zoom, each	Lyons Maid	46.0	0.3	10.0	0.5	n/a
Zucchini: *see Courgettes*						

All amounts given per 100g/100ml unless otherwise stated

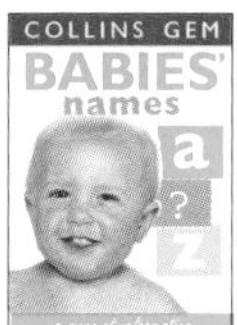
COLLINS GEM
BABIES'
names
a
?
z

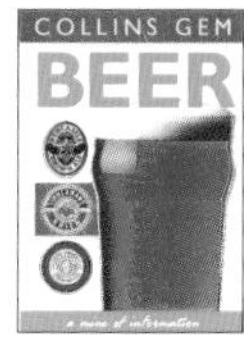
COLLINS GEM
BEER

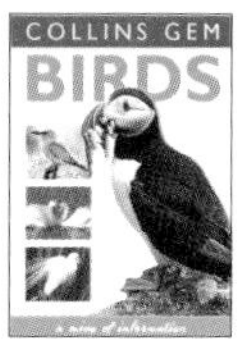
COLLINS GEM
BIRDS

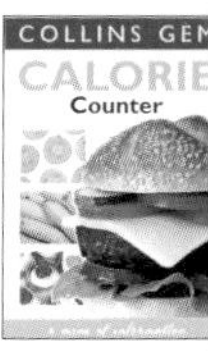
COLLINS GEM
CALORIE
Counter

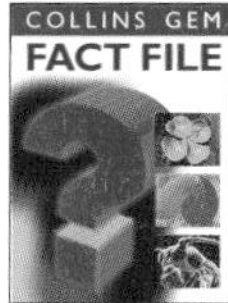
COLLINS GEM
FACT FILE

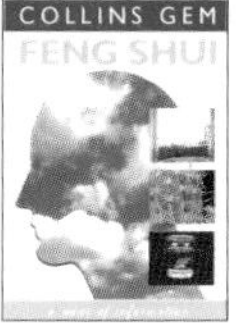
COLLINS GEM
FENG SHUI

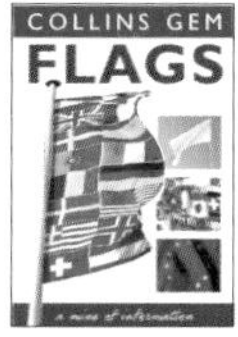
COLLINS GEM
FLAGS

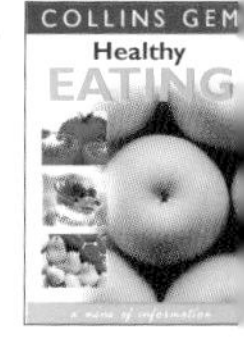
COLLINS GEM
Healthy
EATING

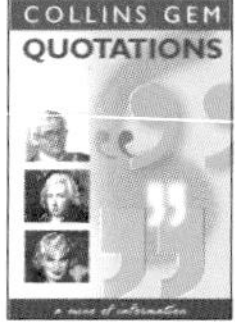
COLLINS GEM
QUOTATIONS

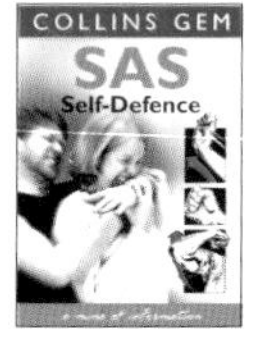
COLLINS GEM
SAS
Self-Defence

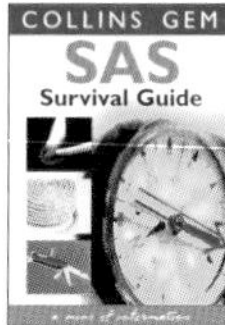
COLLINS GEM
SAS
Survival Guide

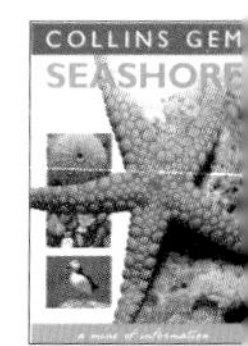
COLLINS GEM
SEASHORE

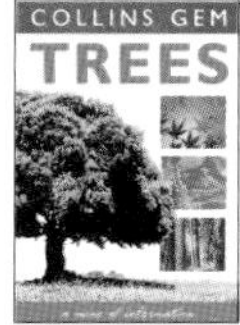
COLLINS GEM
TREES

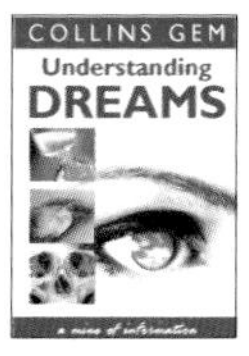
COLLINS GEM
Understanding
DREAMS

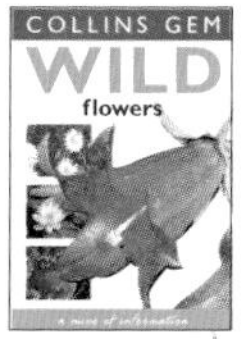
COLLINS GEM
WILD
flowers

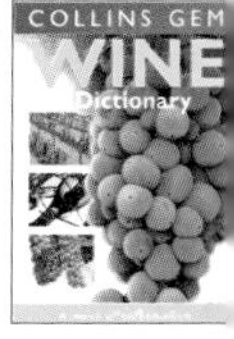
COLLINS GEM
WINE
Dictionary